Pilates Space

THE WORKBOOK FOR INSPIRED ENTREPRENEURS
NICOLA CONRATHS-LANGE AND JENS LANGE

Published by:

Logokinesis Publishing™

805 Third Street

Ann Arbor, MI 48103

USA

Info@logokinesis.com

www.logokinesis.com

Guest Writers: Holly Furgason and Amy Burke

Printed in the United States of America

First printing: 2005

ISBN: 0975506927

Library of Congress Control Number: 2005901686

Cover and text layout: Interkinetic Creative Group™

Cover photograph: Jens Lange

For Claudette

About This Book

-->

"*Pilates Space* is a must-have for any Pilates teacher who owns, or aspires to own, a studio. No Pilates certification will equip you with the information you need to succeed in business. This book provides a unique blend of marketing and industry insights as well as techniques in psychological programming that you will not find anywhere else. We are proud to count Niki as a member!"

—Bernard Slede, President, NAMASTA, North American Studio Alliance

"*Pilates Space* is THE road map for building your mind-body sanctuary. Nicola Conraths-Lange has incredible insight into the inner workings of instruction and ownership, and she puts her ideas together simply and elegantly."

—Kristopher D. Bosch, D.P.T., A.T.C., Dane R. Burke, P.T., A.T.C., Gerald N. Morigerato, B.S., B.A., Cofounders, Northstar Pilates Solutions, LLC

"Niki's first book had a wealth of information that spring-boarded many ideas and solutions. I was hoping for more and here it is! All Pilates junkies owe it to themselves to read her books. We are not alone. It has inspired me to do something about those nagging things that never seem to get addressed. What a gift!"

—Lynette Rasmussen, PT, University of Michigan Spine Program

Disclaimer

Because there is always some risk involved, the author/publisher specifically disclaims any liability, loss, or damage caused or alleged to be caused by this book and accepts no responsibility for omissions or inaccuracies in this book. This includes any adverse effects or consequences resulting from suggestions, procedures, and preparations in this book. Please do not use the book if you are unwilling to assume the risk. Consult your physician or health professional before starting any type of physical activity.

This publication is designed to provide accurate information with regard to the subject matter. It is sold under the understanding that the publisher and authors of this book are not engaged in rendering any legal, accounting, or other professional services. If legal advice or other expert assistance is needed, the services of a competent professional should be sought.

Trademarks in this book are used under license:

Franklin Method™

GYROTONIC®

GYROKINESIS®

Interkinetic Creative Group™

Logokinesis™

Northstar Pilates Solutions™

Pilates Method Alliance®

PMA®

PILATESfoundation® UK Limited

Polestar Pilates Education™

STOTT® Merrithew Corporation

STOTT PILATES™ Merrithew Corporation

Yamuna Body Rolling™

Contents

About the Authors

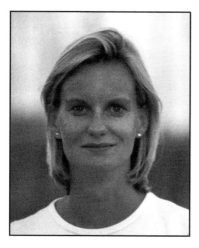

Nicola Conraths-Lange

Nicola Conraths-Lange was born "feet first" and always wanted to dance. She sees herself as a global nomad, following her parents first to Geneva, Switzerland, and then to Rome, Italy, where she grew up.

Dance and movement have been a part of her life since she took her first ballet lesson at the age of five. After a few years of performing with several dance companies and independent projects, she suffered a severe lower back injury which brought her career to an abrupt stop. Still limping and fearful of a future life as an invalid, and with no formal education, she embarked on an exciting venture as an event manager. She toured through Europe with rock groups such as the Rolling Stones, Bon Jovi, Janet Jackson, and Phil Collins, utilizing her languages and organizational skills.

After meeting her future husband Jens, she took a leap and moved to the United States where she avidly pursued bachelor's and master's degrees in communication. At the same time, Pilates came into her life, and amazed at the impact it had on her still hurting body, she decided to certify as a STOTT PILATES™ instructor. Nicola is an instructor teacher for Carolyne Anthony's Center for Women's Fitness, specializing in prenatal and postpartum rehabilitation programs, and is featured in several videos of the center. Her company, Logokinesis, offers workshops, counseling, and teaching advice for teachers in Europe and the United States. Both her books *Survival Skills for Pilates Teachers* and *Pilates Space* are centered on aspects of healthy teaching. She regularly presents at national and international Pilates and dance medicine conferences and has been published in both academic and non-academic journals.

Nicola's future plans include completing her PhD in Performing Arts Studies at Brunel University in London. She currently lives and teaches in Ann Arbor, Michigan, and is an adjunct professor of dance and Pilates at Wayne State University.

Jens Lange

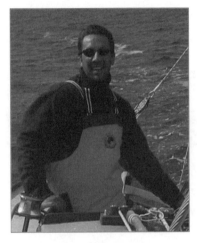

Jens Lange is a long-time automotive professional who works for Freudenberg-NOK in sales and marketing. He completed his MBA at the Hamburger Wirtschafts-Academie in Hamburg, Germany and started out working as a controller for the Board of Phoenix Automotive in Hamburg. Jens moved to the US in 1998 and worked for 3 years as an international program manager, which eventually brought him back to Europe in 2001. After 2 years, he and Nicola went back to the US to follow up on seeds planted some years back, eventually leading to the Logokinesis project.

Jens helped Nicola launch her first Pilates studio in Hamburg, negotiating with equipment manufacturers, shipping companies, and tax experts, and booking sessions with every single studio in the city to check out the competition. He took meticulous notes about each instructor, the environment, the equipment, and the way he was treated. Five years down the line, he sold the Hamburg studio, revamped and designed two additional spaces, and dismantled and reconstructed various pieces of equipment about a dozen times. He is the executive director of Logokinesis Publishing and cowrites and markets Nicola's books. He organized and laid out two manuals for the Center for Women's Fitness in Ann Arbor, Michigan. Jens has a talent for movement photography, is a computer whiz, and is a genius with numbers. In other words, he was born to marry a Pilates teacher.

Today, he is not only working in the automotive industry and the mind-body field with Logokinesis, but he also restores and maintains wooden boats.

Holly Furgason

Holly Furgason comes from a dance background and completed her Bachelor of Dance Arts at the University of Michigan. She began learning about mind-body fitness as a way to strengthen her dance technique. Over the years, her role in mind-body fitness grew from being a Pilates student to being an avid instructor and researcher who is deeply invested in further understanding movement.

Holly began teacher training in STOTT PILATES™ at Equilibrium in Bloomfield Hills, Michigan, and than became an apprentice trainer at The Movement Center in Ann Arbor, Michigan where she worked with Nicola Conraths-Lange. Currently, she is continuing her STOTT PILATES™ education in San Francisco.

At the University of Michigan, Holly's knowledge of aesthetics broadened into the realm of design. Her understanding of form both from movement and visual perspectives has been informed by her professional work as a graphic and Web designer. In 2003, she founded Interkinetic Creative Group™, a full-service graphic and Web design company that specializes in design for the mind-body fitness industry.

In 2004, she was awarded a scholarship to pursue a Master of Fine Arts in Dance at Mills College. Her focus is on choreography, interdisciplinary performance, and dance conditioning through various mind-body fitness modalities.

She is passionate about her work as a Pilates instructor, graphic designer, and choreographer. Holly is dedicated to movement, both visceral and tangible.

Amy Burke

Amy Burke earned her A.B. in philosophy and linguistics from the University of Michigan. While completing her undergraduate degree, she worked as a linguistics research assistant on the Michigan Corpus of Academic Spoken English and held several positions teaching English as a second language—from tutoring a high school English teacher in a small village in Ecuador to holding workshops for graduate students studying abroad at the University of Michigan. She also studied dance and performed in both university and independent projects.

Amy's academic endeavors have taken her around the world. She studied language and literature at the University of Edinburgh and linguistics at York University in Toronto, Canada, and she was invited to present her undergraduate linguistics thesis at a conference on researching and applying metaphor in Tunis, Tunisia.

Amy went on to earn her MPhil in philosophy from University College London, where she focused on the philosophy of language and science. She currently does legal research for an intellectual property firm in San Francisco as well as various writing and editing projects. She is inspired by people like Nicola, Jens, and Holly who take the initiative to create, and she has been thrilled to take part in the Logokinesis publications.

Foreword

When we saw Nicola Conraths-Lange present at the 3rd Annual International Conference hosted by Polestar Pilates Education, we knew right away there was something very special about her. She had the perfect blend of confidence, articulation, and humor in sharing her research with the audience. And who in attendance could ever forget the core musculature after her demonstration using pieces of flex bands, a thong, and an unsuspecting male volunteer!

Pilates Space is the perfect follow-up to Nicola's first book, *Survival Skills for Pilates Teachers*. Nicola once again delves into the issues that are fundamental, yet often go unaddressed. She discusses the business side of our profession and how to discover success within it—covering everything from structuring a business to legal issues to finding the right location for your space.

Owning your own studio makes you, as Nicola describes so well, "wear many hats." You are often owner, manager, practitioner, accountant, cleaner, and more. Balance is the key to success, and Nicola and Jens give us some great guidelines for starting and maintaining a successful mind-body business while preserving sanity, health, and a personal life. While very informative about all of the aspects of structuring a studio, *Pilates Space* is also a great self-assessment tool.

Pilates Space is not just for the Pilates teacher contemplating his or her own studio. Rather, it is for all mind-body professionals—yoga teachers, Feldenkrais practitioners, physical therapists, and personal trainers—to use as a road map to bring their dreams of owning a space to life. Our goal is the same: to make a positive impact on our clients and our communities by realizing our dreams of becoming inspired entrepreneurs.

Thank you, Nicola and Jens, for so eloquently guiding us in our journeys to finding the perfect space!

—Kristopher D. Bosch, D.P.T., A.T.C., Dane R. Burke, P.T., A.T.C., Gerald N. Morigerato, B.S., B.A., Cofounders, Northstar Pilates Solutions, LLC

Introduction

Pilates Space means different things to different people. The concept of space involves the connections between people, things, and processes. Space imposes a universal order. Speaking about, creating, enhancing, shaping, and balancing space in the body is something we think about a lot as Pilates instructors and movement teachers. The concept of space can also relate to mental freedom, the notion of time and how we use it, and financial independence.

We need space in order to grow. We need space for our relationships to be fueled. We need space to do work that is meaningful to us. We need space to regroup and space to give. For Pilates teachers, space has meaning. To our clients, the space we provide, be it mental, physical, emotional, or environmental, is valuable—and it all starts with a room.

This book started taking shape when I realized that several Pilates teachers were all asking me the same question: "What do I need to know to make my Pilates studio successful?" My short answer is that you need to be healthy, you need to be optimistic, you need to care, and you need to plan.

After only five years in the industry, I moved countries twice and started from scratch three times. I also visited Pilates studios (small and large) across the globe—from the United States to Europe to South Africa—to get the "vibe" and distill just which elements make a studio a successful oasis for growth and which do not.

The very fact that we chose mind-body fitness as a career says something about how we will run our businesses. We care for people, and care is an element that money can't buy; it has to emanate from us and will come through in our teaching environments.

A word of caution, though: If you are dreaming about the "big studio," we hope this book will make you consider the pros of running a small family business. Large studios demand a huge amount of work from the owner. Very often, the additional financial and physical drain takes its toll very quickly and turns the very thing you love, doing and teaching Pilates, into an "office job." Too much space creates restriction. The balance is not quite right.

This book is for people who want to have their cake and eat it too. It is for teachers like me who enjoy having a life outside the studio, want to spend time with family and friends, love to travel, and want to keep it that way. Our formula is to start small, build a work schedule that fits your lifestyle, care for your client relationships, and care for yourself.

This manual guides you through the many practical issues that you need to consider before venturing out on your own. The worksheets and checklists at the end of each chapter will make this book a highly personal affair. Write, draw, scribble—do anything that will help you be clear and aware of your needs.

The first chapters ask you to assess your need for change, to visualize the future of your studio, to do some soul searching. Let your inspiration be your guide! Then we will look at communication etiquette. How should you plan for leaving your current job? What is the best way to tell the world that you are going to become a Pilates entrepreneur? Easy formulas will help you prepare and make the transition from employee to owner smoothly and without conflict. Creating common ground with everyone who will be affected by your decision is critical for a successful practice. You want all the good energy you can get.

Chapter 3 presents different options for running your Pilates studio. Are you thinking about a partnership? Which risks are involved? How do you draft a contract, and which elements do you need to discuss with the other owner of your space? Amy Burke introduces some common legal issues in our profession in Chapter 4, interviewing an expert in the field to give you an overview of things you may want to ask an attorney or attempt to do on your own. Jens Lange discusses finances, budgeting, and options for doing it more cheaply as well as things to watch out for when hunting for a space in Chapters 5, 6, and 7. After that, we propose formulas for pricing your classes and will have you build your own schedule with tips and advice on making the most of your time in Chapters 8 and 9, respectively. Holly Furgason will help you promote your space in Chapter 10, covering logos, flyers, advertisements, and how to create your studio's identity. Finally, Chapter 11 talks about the art of pacing and how it helps you get clients in the door and keep them coming back over and over again.

Always remember that Pilates instructors change people's lives for the better. Good teachers have a lot more to offer than a workout. This comes with responsibility. We must take care of ourselves so we can give to others.

So, let's get started doing business the Pilates way. Enjoy.

Inspired Entrepreneurship

CHAPTER ONE

Pilates is a mind-body fitness activity. The mind-body fitness approach is based on the belief that our wellbeing and health originate from a state of physical and mental balance. Balance requires optimal interplay of strength and flexibility, a concept not just applicable to exercise but to our outlook on life as well. It is a foundation for the way we see our bodies and the world. This is why I consider Pilates to be a philosophy—its principles will influence any other type of activity you pursue. Believing that balance is a skill worth striving for requires a specific type of endurance that is much different from directing our energies toward competitive endeavors. We want to look at the bigger picture but also need to attend to our business's alignment, musculature, and power. We also need to know where our weaknesses lie and devise a strategy to tackle them. Pilates entrepreneurs are more than mere business owners. Entrepreneurs have innovative ideas and the zest to pursue them. They take educated risks. They have a clear mission and purpose. They care. As Pilates teachers, we are operating in a complex way: caring for a living, accepting money for care, and keeping feelings of care alive on daily basis. This is not an easy job.

A balanced combination of adventurous spirit, lots of humor, and good planning is the key ingredient of a successful mind-body business.

The recent interest in mind-body fitness is remarkable indeed. Even five years ago, nobody could have predicted that Pilates would become one of the fastest-growing fitness trends of the new millennium. How did this shift come about?

After the group aerobic wave of the 1980's, in which working out was a communal affair and had to involve cardiovascular activity, the 1990's changed our approach to fitness. We wanted to balance, not just to build muscle. We needed calm and quiet to juxtapose our hectic work schedules. We discovered "homemade" wellness that was suddenly accessible to all social classes and not just reserved for the Hollywood stars.

Stores are full of aromatherapy oils for home use, salts and creams, massage balls, yoga mats, eye pillows—many things that were definitely not mainstream just a few years ago. Pampering yourself is okay; in fact, it is finally making its way into our lives as a necessity. Hurray!!

The mind-body boom has catapulted the Pilates method to the forefront of a fast-growing industry. The Pilates Method Alliance®, a not-for-profit professional organization dedicated to preserving the work of Joseph and Clara Pilates, estimated that in the year 2000, 1.7 million Americans had taken at least one Pilates class. In 2001, this number grew to 2.4 million, and in 2002, an amazing 4.7 million Americans had been exposed to the method. *Pilates Style* magazine, a publication that is geared exclusively toward mind-body practitioners, suggests that an astonishing 11 million Americans are now hooked on Pilates.

Oprah recently brought Pilates into millions of homes, demonstrating exercises on the Cadillac and Reformer. Patricia Patrick, one of my colleagues and an instructor in an athletic club, was amazed. "Niki, I could not believe it. I have been teaching Pilates in this club to a select group of clients for four years. None of the fitness trainers were ever interested in finding out more about it. Now Oprah put it on her show, and I am inundated with requests from my colleagues."

What better time to open a studio than now? Admittedly, there probably isn't. And still, people will bombard you with advice and challenging questions: "Pilates is a popular trend. But will it last? What will you do when it is over?"

Here is my candid opinion: **Pilates will last because it works.** It's as simple as that.

Whether individual teachers are going to last, and whether your studio will be here five years from now, depends on you. To start your business with the best possible foundation, there are key questions to consider. At the end of each chapter, there will be a worksheet that will prompt you to answer those questions for yourself. I am asking you to consider the worksheet questions thoroughly and dig deep. Your answers will later develop into the backbone of your business and make things absolutely clear for you. You are likely to refer to them over and over again.

The first set of issues has to do with you and your unique set of skills. Ask yourself:

Do I have a "people-friendly personality"?

As you are considering running your own Pilates space, it is pretty much a given that you enjoy teaching and have an interest in people. For your future job as a Pilates entrepreneur, it is important to realize that being open, friendly, and okay with people is probably not enough. I am asking whether people deeply interest you. If you answer "yes," then you are the kind of person who sits in a restaurant and can barely concentrate on the conversation at your own table because you are busy watching the people scene. You get energized by human interaction, not drained by it. You like to touch and be touched. You don't mind being a confidante as well as an honest discussion partner. You are good even with people you don't like. Human interaction is a driving force in the Pilates space owner's life.

This is important and takes a moment of self-reflection. Are you ready to interact with six to eight clients per day, finish your final class in a good mood, and be ready for more? And after such a day, will you happily keep the interaction going with family and friends? Think about it. You will make yourself and those around you very unhappy if the answer to this is anything other than a definite "Yes! I do."

Do I have a partner, family, and friends who support me?

Running a small business effectively and with low overhead means that you have to wear many hats. You will be responsible for scheduling, accounting, mending the equipment, returning phone calls, cleaning the space, shopping for water and snacks, ordering merchandise, designing flyers, and communicating basic studio events. If a fuse blows, who will fix the lighting? If your space needs renovation, who will be in charge? If you are late, who is going to pick up the kids from school?

Well, as I am sure you know already, the people you love are indispensable. Be clear upfront. Tell them that this is a team effort and you need them. You will be surprised how much pride your family and friends will take in your business if you want to share it with them.

Is this the right time in my life to start my own business?

Have you fulfilled other dreams? Will your commitments in other areas of your life interfere with running a Pilates studio? Will you be able to commit the time it will take to nurture and grow your studio without overextending your resources?

What are my values and how can they be integrated into my business?

If your values are related to social issues or religious activities, you may want to look at those and find a way to integrate what you do with what you believe in. Determining what means something to you and spending some of your time giving to it will make your work much more meaningful and rewarding.

In my studio, we like to help dancers. They are usually not in the position to afford private lessons but can benefit from them enormously. My need to help dancers is linked to my history of being a dancer and getting injured. I value artists and seek to help them. Just as those values enhance my business, your values should enhance yours.

Am I ready to accept the consequences of my choice to own a studio?

Every choice has a consequence. Will you have to set something aside that you enjoy in order to give your business the attention it needs?

Which fears to I need to confront?

Fears are natural, and opening a studio may well give you a couple of sleepless nights. The Dalai Lama says: "There is no point in worrying about things. You can either do something about them or you can't. Worrying does not change the outcome." For me, this concept relates to energy. It takes so much energy to start something by ourselves, to believe in our capabilities enough to take the first step and the thousands that follow in order to complete a goal. The last thing we need is negative energy induced by fear.

Do I have the best education my money can buy?

For a method to work, all the pieces need to fit together. This means that as a new business owner, a top education should be your main priority. There are about eight large Pilates organizations (all members of the Pilates Method Alliance®) that have subscribed to stringent guidelines for the education of their teachers. The Alliance is working hard to make teaching Pilates a federally accredited profession. For an in-depth discussion on this topic, see *Survival Skills for Pilates Teachers*. For now, you and you alone have the power to decide how well-educated you care to be. Every penny, minute, and ounce of effort will be worth it.

Once new teachers have gone through a certification process and suddenly realize just how much is involved in handling clients, many are unsure about how they fit into the grand scheme of teaching Pilates. "How do I know if I am good enough?" is a question that comes up a lot for new trainees.

No need to worry. All you need is the courage to take the time you need to do extensive research and assess your background.

Are you considering Pilates as a career change? Have you spent much of your life being an accountant or a teacher, but have an interest in exercise and just love what Pilates has done for you? Are you just about ready for a big change that will give new direction to your life? These are common scenarios. Many women and men of the baby-boom generation are in the same boat. It's not about the money or the recognition. It's about doing something with your life that you truly enjoy. Turning a hobby into a profession may be your dream. A Pilates studio is a great opportunity to do just that.

Maybe your situation is different. Are you a physical therapist who is bored with the paperwork and the bureaucracy of it all? Are you a dancer who is looking for a movement-related profession, hoping to help dancers, gymnasts, or other artists achieve peak performance? Do you come from a fitness background, and did Pilates make you reconsider everything you ever thought you knew and believed in?

Any of these scenarios is perfectly acceptable; just keep in mind that the time frame for each will be different. Most Pilates organizations will have a comprehensive and an intensive certification track. The comprehensive track takes more time to complete, since you must familiarize yourself with the teaching and assimilation of movement techniques, and all the anatomical theory that lies behind them. Watching experienced educators and completing many apprentice hours is key.

The intensive track is usually faster paced because it assumes that students already know a lot of basic information. The emphasis in intensive courses is placed on exercises and modifications. People in these courses will have had considerable experience working with and looking at the body, which is essential in the profession of teaching Pilates.

Regardless of which track you choose, a good education will give you the following skills, which are essential for running your own show safely and competently. It will require you to spend a considerable amount of time getting familiar with the Pilates principles and exercises. A final test assessing your skills, a practical teaching demonstration, and apprentice hours should be part of a good teacher training program. It will provide you with the necessary anatomical information to make safe choices, considering the mental, physical, and emotional state of your client in establishing a training program. It will train you to master and experience the method on your own body, to the extent that it is safe and beneficial for you to do so. It will provide you with information on the needs of special populations, suggesting modifications for specific injuries or conditions, stressing the difference between your work and that of a physical therapist or a doctor. It will offer professional development options on a regular basis so that you can keep up with new trends and refresh your knowledge of the syllabus.

A top-notch education is especially crucial when you live in an area where there are a lot of Pilates studios already. Your expertise will correlate with the success of your studio. I suggest that you seek apprenticeship opportunities before you venture out on your own. A good reputation is priceless, but it comes with time. Don't rush. Your intuition will tell you when the time is right to go solo.

If you are planning to open a studio in the middle of nowhere, however, things are a little different. Can a Pilates studio really work in a community where nobody has even heard about it?

Yes, it can. Sophie Hunter, a newly certified Pilates teacher, is ready to open a studio in Pinckney, Michigan. The town is very small. The "downtown" essentially consists of one street, and there is no other studio, gym, or fitness facility for miles. Sophie has years of experience as a personal trainer, but has fallen in love with Pilates. She knows everybody in her town and has connections through the local schools, her church, and her family. Her husband is on board, supporting her emotionally and financially. Her education choice is one of the best in the industry. She has charisma, and is open and easy to talk to. This is a great situation, and I have no doubt in my mind that the studio will be a hit. When personality, family support, and expertise come together, it's a win-win situation.

Your personality is your foundation, your family and friends are your cornerstone, and your education is your toolbox. Never compromise on these essential elements. If one of these elements falters, your space is at risk.

WORKSHEET: READY OR NOT?

Why am I seeking change?

1.

2.

3.

4.

5.

This is the right time to open a studio because...

1.

2.

3.

4.

5.

Who will be affected by my decision (family, employer, friends)?

1.

2.

3.

4.

5.

Who are my greatest supporters?

1.

2.

Due to the financial, physical, and mental investments I am about to make, what will I have to sacrifice for a while?

1.

2.

3.

WORKSHEET: READY OR NOT?

Which values do I bring to my studio?

1.

2.

3.

4.

5.

Am I confident that I know enough and have had the right education? Here are five reasons why:

1.

2.

3.

4.

5.

Communication Etiquette for New Studio Owners

CHAPTER TWO

When I opened my first studio, I attempted to do formal research. In Germany, where I lived and worked at the time, it is very important to do "proper" research. Germans are down to earth, like to discuss pros and cons endlessly, and are very likely to dismiss a potential idea unless:

- There is no risk involved.

- The venture is very conventional.

You can probably tell that I was annoyed at the inspiration-killing comments of my compatriots.

In the beginning, when the Pilates space idea is still blooming in your head or you catch yourself bringing it up with your partner or best friend, your vision is your capital and motivator. Starting a business is not a purely solo effort; you will need all the help you can get from people you trust. The process of interacting with people on a one-on-one basis is called "interpersonal communication." Julia Wood, author of *Relational Communication* says that interpersonal communication can be seen as a "generative process that creates understandings between people, defines relationships and identities, composes rules for interaction, and establishes the overall climate of intimacy." When used constructively, timely and effective communication can turn a good idea into a productive reality. Used destructively, it can kill a potentially fantastic vision in its infancy. Communication is a process, so it never really comes to an end; it needs to be renegotiated over and over again. Much like life itself, no two days are alike in terms of the way we interact with people and the types of experiences we have when discussing important news.

Your communication effort is likely to develop in stages. Treat your "baby idea" with the utmost care. Try and meet up with the right people, depending on the goal of each stage of communication. Trust your intuition—sometimes our best friends are not the best ones to talk to about new ideas. Pick someone who has vision and likes to dream.

The Seeding Stage

Picture this: A woman dreams about immigrating to Canada. She has been to Canada several times and loves the people, the climate, the outdoors... you name it. Canada is for her. To whom she communicates her idea in this "blossoming stage" may make or break a potentially great opportunity. Communication is critical at this point.

I divide people to talk to (or rather [not] to talk to...) into two categories: dreamweavers and dreamkillers. Dreamkillers are those people who never create anything but choose to make it their full-time jobs to destroy everybody else's ideas. Dreamweavers are used to taking dreams seriously, realizing that it is the dreaming process that is important, not necessarily the outcome. Dreaming is mental Pilates training.

If our Canada aficionado talks to a dreamkiller, she will have no answers to all the ruthless practical questions the dreamkiller will ask her. She will leave the conversation upset, and her confidence and happiness will have taken a blow.

If she meets a dreamweaver instead, her dream will be enriched by the experiences of another person who is able to visualize and discuss dreams without demanding answers to tough questions. In other words, she will able to speak freely without feeling obligated to act on her dreams. Personally, and to my husband's chagrin, I practice dreaming up ideas often. I believe that it takes just as much training and talent to generate ideas as it does to trim them down and make them workable in reality. If I only practice the "killing," then my ideas will start to fade. I may even end up a dreamkiller myself, spending my days criticizing other people's efforts.

Here is a real-life scenario showing how dreamkillers and dreamweavers practice interpersonal communication:

You say:	Dreamweaver says:	Dreamkiller says:
I have this dream I keep thinking about. I want my own Pilates studio.	A studio! What fantastic idea!	A studio? Are you crazy?
I think I have enough experience to make it work, but of course I am a little worried.	I am sure you will be fully booked in a heartbeat. Positive. Just do it.	Who on earth is going to come to take lessons from you?
I wonder if the timing is right...	This is prefect timing—the economy may not be booming, but you have so much energy and I will help you get it all started! When are we shopping for furniture?	This is terrible timing. The economy is bad. Hundreds of people are out of work. I mean thousands of people are out of work. No, millions of people are out of work...
I have been thinking about the interior, all airy, warm, and calm.	What color shall we paint the walls? Sage green, yellow—oh, you have to have candles.	What interior? You don't even have the money, or a space, or equipment. I can't believe you are even thinking about this stuff now!

Oh! Just writing about dreamkillers' communication efforts makes me feel drained and sad. In fact, Jens and I recently told a family member that we writing a second book and got a perfect dreamkiller reply: "Who the hell is going to read it?" What encouragement... What ever happened to "Congratulations—I think this is amazing"? We talked to the wrong person.

So, avoid dreamkillers in the seeding stage; they will be brought onboard when your project is more developed and you are able to answer all their questions relating to finances, business plans, and contracts in the blink of an eye. In the seeding stage, you want to talk to optimists who are entrepreneurs themselves. Keep in mind what people do to us when they belittle or crush our dreams. I avoid these personalities unless I am well on my way in undertaking a project.

Dreamkillers are fabulous for your business during the blossoming stage, when you need criticism from every corner to make your space successful in the real world.

Blossoming Stage

Be aware that entrepreneurship is something most people dream about, but few have the courage to realize. By the time you communicate your plans to friends and family, you have done much of the psychological groundwork on your own. And yet it is a little frustrating when you break the news expecting excitement and all you get is: "You are leaving your job? Have you thought about this? The economy is so bad right now." The state of the economy is an all-time favorite excuse to avoid venturing into something new, no matter if there is growth or hardship.

People will tell you that your plans are crazy—even people who you really value and love. You need to help them understand what exactly you are planning to do and give them a roadmap of stages. At this point, you should limit those conversations to people you trust; the last thing you need is for your employer to hear about you leaving way before the time is right to go.

In the blossoming stage, you will gather support from your family and friends. You will start looking at the paper and scan advertisements for space rentals. When you go shopping, your eyes will be magically drawn to nice colors of paint or furniture or equipment that you may like to buy. You will start to decorate your space in your head; the blueprint turns colorful and becomes a little bit closer to reality. Slowly, things fall into place: Once you sign a lease, the moment for breaking the news about your dream has come.

--- ➤

Tell it like it is!

Many teachers I have spoken to are fearful of the encounters they will have with their current employers. Where, when, and how to tell them? The scenario described below is middle of the road. You have worked and possibly trained in this studio for a good amount of time, and you respect your employer and are grateful for what he or she had to offer, but you are ready to move on. The foundation here is one of mutual respect.

For this kind of a talk, I would pick a place outside the studio where your roles of employer and employee are not as clear cut. Pick a neutral place; take your employer out to lunch. Make the appointment ahead of time and announce that you have some major changes going on in your life that you would like to share AND (note this carefully!) that you would like some advice. Approach the situation from a mentorship angle and keep the following in mind when you prepare for your meeting:

- All the fears that you may have as a new entrepreneur your employer has probably experienced as well.

- The only difference here is that your employer will have fears regarding you and your role in his or her business.

- In order to reduce your employer's anxiety, you must make sure that you address and respect those fears.

Typically, employers will worry about the following:

1. Timing

   How quickly do you intend to leave? Does it give your employer enough time to phase you out gradually, without losing face? Ideally, you want your employer to be the godmother (or father) of your new studio. Allow your employer to be proud of you. If the relationship is cordial, you may both find this process to be very rewarding. Avoid communicating your plans in an overly matter-of-fact way. Ask for help and support, and you will get it. There are few things more upsetting for an employer than to hear that competition has developed in his or her own space. You both need to work hard at keeping respect intact. During the meeting, create a line of action that helps your old workplace prepare itself for life without you. Try to keep this timeline reasonable for both you and your employer, preferably between two and four weeks.

2.   Where will your studio be located?

Proximity creates competition automatically. I would try, for the sake of your relationship with your employer, to avoid setting up shop in his or her backyard.

3.   Clients

Will you take action to take your clients with you? This is a very sensitive issue, but it needs to be addressed. Ask your employer how he or she would like to handle this. You may be putting yourself at risk if you tell existing clients about your new studio. Generally speaking, if your relationship with your employer is good, he or she will know that some clients will leave to follow you. It is the nature of client-instructor relationships that clients will be loyal to their instructors. They would rather work with you in the phasing-out stage, gradually reducing their hours with you and being introduced to a new teacher, than have you leave abruptly. See Chapter 4 for more details.

In the Hamburg studio where I worked before going out on my own, my employer caught a teacher who was planning to leave stealing all client information that she had accumulated in 15 years. This is a horrible thing to do!

Address these issues candidly during the meeting. Ask your employer how he or she got started. Take notes. Make your employer feel valued. Typically, the hardest scenario is going to be the one where you are one of a few teachers in a small, privately-run studio. If you work in a big gym and teach group classes, you can probably keep that job and move on easily. Your client base and your employer's client base in that situation may be so different that there is no real competition.

Once you have told your employer, the process of detachment begins. At times this can be difficult; you will not have your old role anymore. Be cordial, punctual, and professional until the very last day. You have plenty of work to do in your time off!

Ugly situations?

In my experience, most detachment processes have worked quiet well. On the other hand, we would be naïve to think that there are no pitfalls in the process of leaving your employer. The scary word here is "lawsuit."

While completing my research for this book, I have spoken to a few teachers who experienced a lot of trouble that resulted from leaving their jobs. They agreed that it is wise to refrain from mentioning to any of your clients that you are planning to open a studio. One teacher who had consulted with a lawyer prior to quitting was told that she could only say that she is planning on remaining active in the same line of work.

Nancy Hodari, owner of the STOTT PILATES™ certification center in Bloomfield Hills, Michigan is not only a teacher and entrepreneur, but a lawyer as well. I asked her about employees' rights and responsibilities when they have signed agreements with their employers. "If the non-compete, non-solicitation provision is fair and does not inhibit a person's ability to make a living, then it is upheld in a court of law," she says. "I am not aware of any instances where they have been litigated, just a few examples of where they were respected." Be sure that you know what your contract with your employer requires of you before you speak to anyone at your current job about your new business.

Usually, it seems that a relationship needs to be under a considerable amount of stress to warrant serious disputes. We are not exactly known to be people who love hurting others—quite the contrary. If you are unhappy with your job for whatever reason, just leave and find a different way to bridge the time between leaving your old job and starting the new studio.

One studio owner who was actually sued by a former employer said: "If you are considering leaving your job, you should always use professional etiquette. However, there are some situations that warrant your immediate removal especially if they are in violation of your ethical and moral standards. In essence, this makes a difficult decision straightforward and easy to make. I have found that there can be a vast discrepancy between an employer's perception of events and the reality of a situation. Although you may attempt to rehabilitate the relationship, there is a threshold as to how much you are personally willing to endure. This point is different for everyone, and once you reach it, change your environment as soon as you possibly can. My advice is to be prepared for the worst because your previous employer may make attempts to slander or even sue you, providing a version of the events that favors him or her. Ultimately, people will make their own decisions based on the information they have. Always remain steadfast and true to your morals, and be the better person. It is what separates us from them, and people will respect you for it."

So, be ready to leave immediately if that seems to be the best option for you.

Blooming Stage

In the blooming stage, things are in place from a communication perspective. You have told everybody about your decision who will be affected by it. So, now it is out with the old and in with the new. In the beginning, you most likely will have no clients! Due to the fact that we identify so much with the work we do, this can cause some anxiety. We have to start from scratch and establish our credibility in our own space. When I opened my first studio, I sat on the Cadillac and could not envision one single person walking in the door. I was so excited when it finally happened that I thought I should pay the client and not vice versa.

It is overly optimistic to rely on your friends to get your studio going in terms of clientele. It is important for your development as a teacher and an entrepreneur to get the first clients in the door without help. Every client who comes in the door and stays will reflect your personal achievement. Your studio will grow and prosper, and the credit will go to you. All your friends and acquaintances will have to be treated as clients as well without special treatment—although some will try and ask for favors.

Mary is a studio owner in the making. She has not even unpacked her equipment yet. The grand opening is fast approaching, but builders are still working on the space. She goes for lunch with a friend who insists on paying. Mary thanks her and says, "Next time it'll be on me!" Her friend says, "Oh don't worry, you can just keep a tab for me at your new studio." Mary is really shocked. "How am I going to make ends meet if all my friends who have offered support hope for discounts?"

When these situations come up, be honest. Tell your friends that you have invested a lot in this studio and are unable to give discounts. If they have something to offer that you need, you may want to consider trading services.

Once those are gone, there are no more discounts. Mary also communicates to her clients that her prices go up every 18 months to account for inflation. These are two great ways to be kind while establishing rules at the same time.

Communicating well helps you create common ground. If you are scared of an encounter, do the following exercise, commonly used by communication coaches for neurolinguistic programming (NLP): Close your eyes and visualize the scene. Picture what you will be wearing, where you will be sitting. Then observe yourself talking from an outsider's position. Analyze whether your points are correctly made, and whether you are clear and concise. Then imagine all the corresponding details about the person with whom you are communicating. If talking to your employer makes you nervous, play out different scenarios of how he or she could react. Role playing is an amazing tool to take the anxiety out of upcoming situations. No matter what happens, you will be prepared and your reactions will be rehearsed. Again, the bottom line is that we need to train for an important event. Just as we wouldn't have a client do the hundreds right off the bat, we should not go into a potentially challenging situation without a proper warm-up.

Communication is about more than just what we tell other people and when. According to Osamo Wiio, communication is inescapable and irreversible. This means that if you do not communicate, it sends a very clear message to people surrounding you: "I am doing my own thing and I don't care about you." Therefore we cannot *not* communicate. We communicate with language, with silence, with our bodies, with our eyes, and with the space we choose to place between ourselves and others. Oftentimes, situations get out of hand without our being aware of the damage we caused. We may think: "But I didn't say or do anything to that person!"

Pick your battles wisely, and consciously direct effort and good energy into communication.

Seeding Stage

Who are three dreamweavers in my community of friends and family?

1. _____

2. _____

3. _____

Who are three dreamkillers in my community of friends and family?

1. _____

2. _____

3. _____

This is my vision for my new studio:

Blossoming Stage

What am I scared of?

1.

2.

3.

4.

5.

What fears can I do something about (e.g., reassure my employer about his or her fear of competition)?

1.

2.

3.

4.

5.

What fears can I not control or make better (e.g., general anxiety about failure or finances)?

1.

2.

3.

4.

5.

Who will I tell about my dream first and when?

1.

2.

3.

Blooming Stage

What are the policies for my studio (e.g., pricing, discount, cancellation)?

1.

2.

3.

4.

5.

I will practice NLP with the following people to prepare for my meetings:

1.

2.

3.

Better Together? Partnerships, Contracts, and Best Friends

CHAPTER THREE

BETTER TOGETHER?

A partnership is a symbiotic relationship; one element is not complete without the other. Many Pilates studios that I have come across in the past have been partnerships at some point. It works well for some, and others claim that they will never do it again. A business partnership is much like a marriage; it even has about a 50% chance of failure within the first two to four years. The primary cause for this failure is poor communication.

Anne Deering and Anne Murphy discuss the growing trend of partnerships at length in their book, *The Partnering Imperative: Making Business Partnerships Work*. They report that partnerships can bring in a 25% higher profit than solo competitors could, but that 70% of joint ventures do not succeed.

The more you know about why partnerships fail, the less likely you will be to "break up" with your partner. Each of the issues listed below is a common reason for tension between partners, according to Camilla Cordell of *Profit Magazine*. I have taken the liberty to rephrase her list for a Pilates context:

1.   Division of Workload

A common problem in partnerships is that one person believes he or she cares more and works more for the business without being rewarded for it. Nancy Hodari, owner of Equilibrium in Bloomfield Hills, Michigan, experienced this firsthand in her studio. "In a partnership, there is always one person who cares more and therefore works more," she says. "At the beginning, you look over it. But after a while it gets to you."

I would suggest that in these instances we pick our battles wisely. If the studio is doing well and your complaints are related to organizational matters, bring them up, talk about possible solutions, and end it then and there. Oftentimes, however, changes in the way your business partner acts may be related to private matters. If that is the case, part of being a partner is caring for the other person and possibly taking over some of his or her job responsibilities for a limited amount of time. This should not become the normal state of affairs.

2.   Lack of Communication

Last month, this issue hit home at the studio I share with my business partner Aimee McDonald. We see each other all day long. "See" is the right word here—not "talk." We communicate through short notes and had not been able to make time to have coffee or lunch with each other in months. After we finally communicated, problems were solved and things were good again. Make time for each other at least once a week.

3. Want your sister to take over?

Family members are important for the functioning of our studio. If I had to call a plumber, painter, or electrician every time something needs fixing in the studio, I would be completely broke. My family and friends are willing to help, and there is no problem in asking them for those kinds of favors.

Problems arise when family members of one of the business partners plan on taking over whole sections of the business. If your partner's younger sister is planning to become a teacher and your partner is enthusiastically making plans for her to join the partnership, how are you going to voice your concerns?

4. We are a Pilates studio. What do you mean you want to teach Gyrotonic®?

Entrepreneurs may have very different visions of where their partnership is headed. A change of direction usually involves investment. If one of the partners is not remotely interested in what you are planning, there is trouble ahead.

My partner Aimee, for example, is a Gyrotonic® pre-trainer. The way her business is going, she will need a second Gyrotonic® Tower soon. She also wants to buy the Jumping-Stretching Board and possibly the Ladder in a few years. I want a second Reformer. We have a problem already because our space is very, very small. Thankfully in our case, the problem is of a logistic nature. We occasionally talk about the possibility of renting a larger space in the not-too-distant future. Plans change and needs change. Communication about our visions ensures that we are on the same page.

5. I don't want to teach Pilates anymore.

If one of the partners wants out because he or she is pursuing other interests, that's okay. The important thing is to do this gradually so that neither partner is pushed into making hasty personal or financial decisions.

By putting things down in writing, we have the greatest possible chance of keeping our friendships intact and our investments protected. If there is no paperwork, you have a very weak leg to stand on if a dispute arises. A partnership is not necessarily legally binding if it is founded on a handshake and a promise. An "out clause" in your partnership contract is a must to avoid harsh consequences.

Depending on which state's laws govern your partnership, certain aspects such as liability, profits, and property will be affected. Check out Chapter 4 for information on business entities and the additional resources at the end of the book for more detailed information.

To lay the proper foundation, take time with your potential partner to create an agreement that addresses at least each of the following basic issues:

- The business name

- Who will sign the lease and what its terms should be

- When the partnership will start and its projected length

- Amount each partner is going to invest and what percentage that is of the whole investment

- Who pays for the equipment and an inventory of who owns what going into the partnership

- Who sets up bank accounts and credit cards for the business and how they will be maintained

- How profits and losses are split

- How new clients are handled and who gets what business

- Ownership of client database

- Costs of running the studio

- Vacation time each partner can take

- Ability to work for other Pilates or exercise-related businesses

- Out clause: what happens if one partner wants out and the procedure for handling a split

This agreement can be anything you want it to be. Just write down what is important to you and compare notes. Make sure to consult a lawyer and an accountant to get advice on forming your partnership before you finalize any decisions, and keep different versions of the agreements you adopt just in case you need them in the future to show how you reached and agreed on the final draft.

Now that we have addressed the main reasons why partnerships fail, it is also good to know that some partnerships work beautifully and are a lot of fun. Working with a partner is energizing—you can share studio-related mishaps (and hopefully laugh about them), and you can have someone you trust ready to cover for you. Advantages of a partnership include:

1. More capital

More people often equal more investment capital to create just the studio you want. Buying equipment and leasing a space requires money. On your own, you may have a harder time convincing the bank to give you a loan or finalizing a rental agreement. Having said that, always be aware that as a partner you not only share the profit but the losses as well.

2. Shared workload

Two people can share tasks that are overwhelming for one person. The key is to split duties equally and respect each other's aptitudes. There is no reason to make one partner do accounting if neither of you is good with numbers. Get an accountant.

3. Tax advantages

There may be some tax advantages when you operate as a partnership rather than as a sole proprietor. Get an expert to walk you and your partner through the tax issues.

Once you have worked through these steps in setting up a partnership, a substantial chunk of time should be devoted to exploring the partners' goals, personalities, and energy levels. The following elements make a partnership worthwhile and enriching. We are leaving the world of cold business facts here and entering a more spiritual domain.

Vision

A common vision is the rhythm that makes you and your partner move together in the grand scheme of things. It is ultimately a mission statement that justifies and gives meaning to who you are and what you would like to accomplish with your studio.

The owners of Northstar Pilates Solutions™ in Buffalo, New York, Kristopher Bosch, Dane Burke, and Gerald Morigerato, are the perfect advocates for partnerships that not only work well and make a business grow, but share a common vision. Kris has just completed his doctorate in physical therapy, Dane is a licensed physical therapist, and Gerry holds a degree in exercise physiology and psychology. All three of them have had the good fortune to work closely with Brent Anderson, Shelly Power, and Marilyn Mardini at Polestar Pilates. Northstar Pilates Solutions opened in early 2004 and offers appointments and classes from 7AM to 7PM on weekdays and on Saturday mornings.

In fact, I first met the "Buffalo Boyz" at the Polestar conference in Miami last year. I was intrigued and impressed. "Wow! Three guys running a Pilates studio. I haven't come across that one before."

Dane, Kris, and Gerry had very similar visions, which make this unusual partnership work so well. I had the opportunity to ask them some questions about their new business.

Niki: When you started your studio, did you verbalize a common goal or vision that you wanted to achieve?

Dane: One of the most startling things that I see with us is sometimes it seems as though we are linked on some other plane. I remember on more than one occasion, Kris and I were working at the same facility (Gerry was at our other location), and we had decided that we should actively start marketing to physicians by creating a PR packet that we could deliver to them. Not two minutes after we were done discussing it, we get an email from Gerry saying that he was thinking that an information packet that was geared toward physicians would be a good way to market our rehab services. This is one of those times where it seems as though we can communicate without talking. Strange but very cool!

Niki: Two of you are physical therapists, and yet you decided to focus your practice completely on Pilates. How did this come about?

Kris: We are all interested in research on Pilates rehabilitation, and feel strongly that our mission is to effect change in the health system as whole and increase awareness of the positive impact Pilates can have in our communities.

Dane: Research is definitely one of our main priorities. Getting private insurance carriers to pay for these services without any reservations requires clinical research, whether qualitative or quantitative, to prove the efficacy of Pilates as a rehab tool. Now mind you, in ten years I hope that battle will be won, but ongoing research will always aid in substantiating our PROFESSION. This is a very important point to make. When I tell people that I am a Pilates instructor, the next question usually is: "Well, what is your real job?"

Niki: Where do your see yourselves ten years from now?

Dane: In ten years, I see us as being a multi-faceted facility that offers Pilates and a variety of mind-body services: Gyrotonic® and Gyrokinesis®, Yamuna Body Rolling™, Franklin Method™, NLP. We all see the value of offering manual therapy techniques to supplement the movement and mind-body integration.

Niki: How do you market your studio?

Kris: Even though we are all physical therapists, we consistently market our studio as "Pilates only." We have a 60/40 split in terms of patient–client distribution. Having said that, all clients, patients, and healthy people alike are private pay. We can work with insurance in some cases, but overall, people come because they are impressed with what we have to offer: one-on-one training for an hour in a strictly Pilates environment.

Niki: Did you think about the type of partnership you were going to have? How did you prepare?

Kris: We did not really think about all the issues with partnership much. We run two spaces. The first one, in an up-and-coming commercial complex (650 ft^2), was a great price, and we just went for it and opened up shop. We also have a room in the downtown hospital that we use.

Niki: Gerry, you have the role of business manager. Does it make sense to divide up roles ahead of time within the organization?

Gerry: As president of this company, it is my job to oversee every facet of the business. Of course, I have delegated certain roles and responsibilities to others, but the overall direction of the business is under my care. I can't over-emphasize the importance of delegating tasks to others. If you believe that you will be able to wear all of the hats of operating a business at once, you are setting yourself up for disaster. Your success will be dictated by your ability to share the workload involved in the process. Who is responsible for what, and who is being held accountable for your actions? Although these roles may overlap at times, it is important that all facets be covered, and that a constant flow of communication is present. Your ability to communicate is critical in determining the success of your business.

Niki: Did you want to be business person?

Gerry: Initially I assumed the role of the "business person" because there really wasn't anyone else to do it. I had limited business experience and realized that I needed to formulate a business plan and utilize all of the resources that I had available to me. There was definitely a learning curve involved in the process. Since my business plan was so well organized, everything worked itself out. Remember there will always be challenges along the way—some you expect, and others you don't expect.

Niki: What are the advantages of a partnership?

KRIS: We have an even split in our business, so there is never any tension regarding who has ultimate power to make decisions. Of course, with more people involved, you will have differing opinions on how to run things at times. But, we have so much common ground and a larger vision regarding what we want to achieve long term that the discussions make us stay grounded. We truly are in this together!

DANE: Being in a partnership definitely is interesting. I grew up in a family with four older brothers, so I had early life lessons in compromise. Compromising is important, especially when all three of us feel so strongly about the success of our business. We all have ideas that we think are important, but compromising and fully supporting the direction we decide to take is what will make us successful.

There will always be differences of opinion, but respecting those differences is something we do well.

The Buffalo Boyz story is a real-life example of what this book advocates: Have a vision, start small, get things going, and then think about expanding.

The Role of Personality

Think about your personality and your partner's. Do they match? Are they diametrically opposite? You don't have to be an energy bomb for your studio to work if you're on your own, but it certainly helps to have the kind of charisma that draws clients in. If your partner has a strong personality, you can be less outgoing and still reap the benefits of having a bustling studio. The trick is to allocate areas of expertise that match your interest levels and skills. Energy bombs are rarely good at numbers. However, skillful account management is crucial for the studio to succeed. Will you be satisfied if you are the one working in the background and the other partner is in the limelight? Decisions should be made together, taking strengths and weaknesses into account. Divide up your areas of responsibility and decide ahead of time what role you will have and how you would like to be rewarded.

Here are just a few examples: Do you want your achievements to be celebrated publicly? Then a party once a year where you invite all your clients, friends, and the press (oh yeah!) will give you the overt appreciation that you need to be happy and feel valued. I am a prime example of a person who needs to feel like a diva once in a while. (Talk to my friends... they may even suggest I need this all the time.) You can give me more money, and I won't really care that much if my work is teaching Pilates in a dungeon to bats. No—pas mois! I like the limelight.

Other people hate being on display and are happiest if their paychecks increase and they get treated to a massage or spa once a year instead of an extravagant party. The bottom line is this: We all need to feel valued, but personality determines how we are measured and rewarded. Paul and Sarah Edwards are the gurus of home businesses. In their book *Working from Home*, they describe ways of working that fit different personalities. This is useful to be aware of from a partnership perspective as well. Basically, workers can be divided into two categories: segregators and integrators.

Segregators are those people who need to have the workplace separate from the home. Work is one thing; private life is another. They also are the ones who will organize a Pilates studio in a segregated manner. When you are planning the studio layout, a segregator may say: "This is where the appointment book goes. This is where the pens go. This is the box for our business cards." A segregator will ideally want a separate office room in the studio. If that is not possible due to space concerns, you need to arrange for a designated area for that person's segregational needs to be satisfied.

If a segregator shares a studio with an integrator, the integrator needs to refrain from doing what he or she does best: mixing. Integrators will disperse planner pages, notes, and schedules all over the studio, lie on the roller as they return phone calls, and think nothing of it to have a client do footwork on the reformer while they make tea.

Combining various elements of life into one feels perfectly natural to an integrator. An integrator who teaches Pilates out of her home, for example, can put a Cadillac in the kitchen and be professional without any problems. A segregator who is forced to work this way will never quite feel comfortable.

Be aware of this issue and discuss it with your Pilates partner so you can plan accordingly.

Energy

In a successful mind-body partnership, both teachers bring good energy to a studio. I don't really care what other criteria listed on a resume I am supposed to look at, but if a person who wants to work in the studio comes through the door, I can't help but immerse myself in his or her aura. Bad energy is hard to balance in a place of mind-body study and training. Good energy, on the other hand, is immediately apparent to clients and other teachers. Good energy is one of the reasons that our studios thrive. The question of energy in a partnership deserves a lot of attention. So how can we best describe such a subjective matter?

A person with good energy looks at life in a positive way. Her walk has energetic zest to it; her posture signals openness and welcome. Her senses are alert, and she shows interest in what surrounds her. When she talks, her voice has highs and lows.

Quite the opposite holds true for people with bad energy.

Kris summed it all up: "We are very lucky in that we have a great working energy between the three of us, which is so pivotal to making a partnership work. We are all like-minded, yet we each bring something unique to the table. Even when there are big decisions or sensitive issues, we are always on the same page that what we are doing is business, and there is never a personal criticism involved. With the three of us, there is never any ego involved either.

"I guess you could say that it is really all about intentions. As long as our intentions are good and we are moving in a direction of beneficence, then good things will continue to happen to us!"

As for the colder, more business-oriented aspects of partnerships, we have seen how researching financing and legalities prior to opening a studio is pivotal for long-lasting success in the real world. Within this frame, chemistry between partners, communication, and a willingness to compromise for a larger vision will ultimately be what makes you happy. Your vision should be larger than life. "I want to have 30 clients 10 years from now" just will not do.

Take Kris, Dane, and Gerry's example: **We want to change the health system so that it embraces mind-body therapies.**

A dreamkiller would say they are completely mad. Dreamweaver that I am, I can't wait for it to happen.

Notes:

WORKSHEET: YOUR PARTNERSHIP

Start by having each partner work on this first section of the worksheet independently.

What do you bring to the business that your potential partner lacks?

1.

2.

3.

What does your potential partner bring to the business that you lack?

1.

2.

3.

Hopefully, you know your potential partner well. In light of what was discussed in Chapter 3, who will be the one who cares more and therefore works more? Why do you think so?

Is there anything in your potential partner's personality that sends you up the wall? What is it?

How will you handle it?

Are you comfortable negotiating a partnership contract?

Is the financial investment into your new studio equally divided between you and your partner? If not, how will it be divided?

Do you feel that your financial investment is fair given your partner's investment?

Do you deeply trust this partnership? If you have doubts, what are they?

WORKSHEET: YOUR PARTNERSHIP

Which role will you play in the partnership? Describe your profesional disposition in your own words.

List some jobs mentioned in this chapter that you would like to take on.

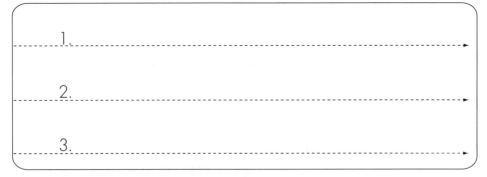

1.

2.

3.

Are there any jobs you want to avoid? List them below.

1.

2.

3.

Now compare your answers to the questions above with your partner's. Take some time to discuss any answers that are new or surprising to either of you. Then complete the next section together.

My jobs will be:

1.

2.

3.

4.

5.

My partner's job will be:

1.

2.

3.

4.

5.

WORKSHEET: YOUR PARTNERSHIP

Our legal advisor is:

Our CPA/tax advisor is:

Decide on a weekly meeting time and place for you and your partner. When and where will it be?

Protecting Your Space

CHAPTER FOUR

AMY BURKE

PROTECTING YOUR SPACE

The stronger the foundation for your new business, the better chance it has to thrive. At this point, you've already considered several factors that will make or break a Pilates studio: your personal needs and desires, how you will communicate with "dreamkillers" and "dreamweavers," and whether you want to enter into a partnership or go into business on your own. Once you have considered these choices carefully, you have laid solid groundwork for the personal and interpersonal aspects of your new business.

Now it's time to think about how to give your Pilates studio a strong foundation from a legal standpoint. This chapter will cover the benefits of seeking legal advice when you open your new studio and what to expect from an attorney. It will also give you tips on how to keep costs down by taking on some of that work yourself.

You may know people who have started and maintained successful Pilates studios without ever setting foot into a law office, and you may prefer to take care of these things on your own as well. However, a little protection can seem invaluable if something goes wrong. What if:

You have just had your first piece of equipment delivered—a brand new Reformer. By the time you and your partner are thoroughly exhausted from trying to move it into the perfect spot in your studio, you slide it directly under the skylight. It's perfect! Your clients will be able to gaze up at the stars or have plenty of natural light in the middle of the day. In fact, you had just spent hours on a ladder cleaning the skylight so that you and your clients could really enjoy it. You leave for the weekend, looking forward to your first private session on Monday. When you return to your studio before your client arrives, you are horrified to find that the seal had been broken around the skylight and the weekend's downpour has damaged your beautiful Reformer. As you are mopping up the water from the hardwood floor that your landlord refinished just before you moved in, your client comes in and slips on the slick entryway, twisting her ankle as she falls.

Now, suppose that you haven't gotten around to forming your business entity or purchasing insurance. Suppose you have no idea what the warranty on your new Reformer is like or where you can find someone to repair it. Suppose you have absolutely no idea what your liability is as far as your lease is concerned—you aren't sure whether it's your responsibility or the landlord's to repair the water-damaged floor. Finally, suppose that your client has had a couple private sessions with you. She hadn't told you about any health problems or that the exercises you did with her were causing her any pain, but she suddenly decides that your work with her has made her weaker and more prone to injury. That evening, you frantically search for a lawyer, but you have no idea how to find someone you can trust. What a mess!

Clearly, this scenario is pretty extreme, but it's meant to show that even a little preparation can go a long way. Keep in mind that even if you're not the type of person who is naturally inclined to take preventative measures, your thoughts on this may change once you actually get started with your own business. A North American Studio Alliance (NAMASTA) survey recently revealed that 84% of mind-body professionals are "somewhat concerned" or "very concerned" about the possibility of a lawsuit.

Consider an alternative to the ill-prepared studio owner described above: Your business entity was properly formed, you have purchased appropriate insurance, you have a well-negotiated lease for your space, you understand all of the agreements you have with your certifying organization and equipment manufacturers, and your clients have all signed the proper releases and information forms. If a client is injured during a session, you are likely to be protected. If your business is very successful in its current location and you don't want your landlord to rent your space to someone else after your first year, you are likely to be protected.

Now, it's natural to associate preventing a problem with the problem itself—who wants to worry about the millions of things that could go wrong? You may wonder whether you really want to spend the money or take the time out of your own busy schedule to make sure you're protected from all of the potential problems that could occur.

This approach, however, is like teaching a brand new Pilates client advanced material without giving her a proper foundation in the basics... not only would she miss out on many of the benefits Pilates has to offer, but she is much more likely to reinforce bad habits and to get injured.

Dealing with the technical business issues now (rather than when disaster strikes) will give you peace of mind, and it will allow you to get the most out of your business relationships and the contracts you enter into. Perhaps most importantly, it will allow you to address potential problems now instead of when they actually happen. Think of it as injury prevention!

The Issues

This chapter will give you an overview a range of potential issues that you may consider as you build your new business. The specific issues that you will need to address in creating a solid legal foundation for your new studio will depend on your individual needs.

This chapter is also for those of you who are worried about spending your initial consultation with a lawyer trying to figure out what issues are most important discuss. The best way to learn about the legal side of business is to ask an expert, and I had the opportunity to interview an attorney who specializes in the field. Not only does he have several mind-body fitness clients and extensive experience in helping their studios grow and remain successful—he also takes Pilates and is a strong believer in its benefits.

Owen Seitel is a partner of Idell Berman Seitel & Rutchik, LLP in San Francisco, California. His practice focuses on both transactions and litigation involving intellectual property and business with an emphasis on legal and business issues of particular concern to those operating in the sports and entertainment industries. Owen is a member of the California State Bar, the San Francisco Bar Association, the American Bar Association Forum on the Entertainment and Sports Industries, and California Lawyers for the Arts. He is also an adjunct professor at the Golden Gate University School of Law, where he teaches courses on intellectual property content licensing.

AMY: In general, what kind of work do you do? Who are your clients?

OWEN: I deal with people who are creators in the broad sense. Obviously, that includes people who are involved in the arts or entertainment. But it also includes people who have ideas and seek to find a way to implement those ideas, and maybe even make money from them. I see art and entertainment as including not only the traditional arts, such as music and film, but also every kind of athletic endeavor—whether it is some kind of choreographed fitness routine like yoga or Pilates or something more freeform like basketball—it is all art to me in that it requires creativity and, if it is good, it will capture an audience, either as passive consumers or active participants. So, I see anyone who's involved in any kind of creative endeavor that has the potential to capture an audience as a great client.

AMY: If a Pilates instructor just wants to open a small studio on her own, why should she see an attorney?

OWEN: First of all, if you're going to open a Pilates studio, you have many of the same issues that any other business will have. As with any other business, before you open the doors you will need to enter into contracts. Typically, your first contract is going to be a lease, and that's a significant contract because it is usually for a period of years and you're going to be bound by that contract whether your business fails or succeeds. Note that I said "You" are going to be bound by that contract, regardless of the success of your business. Most landlords will require that you co-sign or personally guarantee the lease your business enters into. So if you enter into a three-year lease but your business folds after one year, you, personally, will typically be on the hook for the remaining two years of that lease.

You also may have employees or independent contractors working for you, and you should have agreements with them. It is important to have something in writing with those who you work with and for you to ensure that both parties understand their relative obligations and expectations, because not all relationships end well. When an employment or contractor relationship ends it is not uncommon for each of the parties to have divergent recollections of the terms they agreed upon—perhaps the hours of work, the rate of pay, commissions, etc.–so it is important to have a written document, signed by both parties when they are optimistic about the relationship and their heads are cool, laying out these terms.

Your relations with your landlord and those who work with and for you point out one important legal goal in the early stages of your business planning–the need to try to limit your personal liability. The owner of a business usually goes into the start-up process very optimistically (and if you are not optimistic, you should not attempt a new business venture). When someone comes to see me at these early planning stages I often feel bad because I end up playing the role of the grim reaper and showing the client everything that could go wrong. It is not a lawyer's role to paint a rosy picture. Rather, it is the lawyer's role to tap into his or her knowledge and experience of how and why things go wrong and then point out ways in which the client can obviate or alleviate any of those things the best we can.

One of the best ways to avoid personal liability is to form a limited liability entity, typically either a corporation or an LLC, and operate the business through that entity. All states recognize corporations and most if not all states recognize limited liability companies. Basically, what you are doing by creating a business entity is creating another person in the eyes of the law. The entity can then enter into agreements, sue and be sued, open a bank account, etc.

Why do you do that? If someone walks into the studio, slips on a banana peel, and cracks his head open on your floor, ideally his claim is against the entity, not you personally, because it is the entity that operates the business, entered into the lease, and cleans the floor. If it is the entity that operates the business, the injured person couldn't necessarily come after you personally and get a judgment against you that may allow him to take the money in your bank account, your car, your bicycle, or anything else that you own. Rather, he would have to go after the assets of the liable party–the entity–and seek recovery from the bank account and other assets owned by the entity.

There are many scenarios where that liability can arise. Someone could get injured while doing Pilates training, the equipment could fail, etc. This is why, in addition to operating your business through a limited liability entity, you should obtain liability insurance. First, it is likely that your landlord will require that you obtain liability insurance coverage and further require that they be named as an additional insured on your policy. Why is this? Because if someone does get injured by slipping on a banana peel in your studio, he or she is likely to sue not only you, but also the landlord and any other party they can connect to this potential liability. Second, even if the landlord does not require that you carry insurance coverage, you should do so. Liability insurance is a subject that we could go into tremendous detail discussing. Instead, assume that you will need to secure insurance and discuss the issue with your attorney.

Getting back to the lease, if possible, the entity can enter into the lease, and then if you have to break the lease, the worst the landlord can do is sue the entity. However, any time you enter into a lease as a new entity, the landlord is typically going to require that you co-sign the lease or that you personally guarantee the lease. This is because a start-up entity is typically going to have few assets. Most landlords know this, and they will require a backup to make sure that someone is responsible in a back-up position in the event the business fails and the entity dissolves but amounts remain due under the lease. Typically that back-up will be you, personally, but if your assets are not that impressive, it is common that a guarantor with greater wherewithal will be required.

On the other hand, if you're IBM, or possibly a business that has been in existence for a while with a history of some success and some assets, your landlord is more likely to allow your entity to enter into the lease agreement without your personal guarantee.

TIP: If you have friends who rent business spaces, start asking around about prices, realtors, and terms and conditions of commercial leases. It will give you some valuable background for your first few encounters with potential landlords.

AMY: What about the possibility of entering into a residential lease rather than a commercial lease?

OWEN: That's always possible. But the dictates for the market that you're in are going to determine what kind of lease you could get. I would say if you were looking for any kind of rental space in San Francisco in 1997, you weren't going to find it, especially if it were some individual hoping you were going to open a Pilates studio. And then in 2000, you could potentially get a space for one year. Keep in mind, there are pros and cons to a one-year lease. The pro, of course, is that you know the fullest extent of your liability. But if you enter into a one-year lease at a reasonable monthly rent and you find in month 11 that you have a very successful Pilates studio going, you will have to renegotiate your lease. That landlord is going to be observant of your success and see what is going on—he's now in line to extract more money for the lease. On the flip side, if you enter into a long-term lease, you know what you are going to be paying in rent in the future, and, more importantly, you know where your business will be located in the future. So there are pros and cons to both a short-term and a long-term lease. At its shortest, you could get a month-to-month lease. That of course leaves you subject to getting kicked out of your space at the end of every month. That's problematic.

AMY: One issue for Pilates instructors who already work for other studios is how to handle moving out on their own. Nicola has discussed some basic rules of etiquette, such as how to communicate with an employer about such a decision [see Chapter 3]. She suggests speaking candidly about the new business venture, and asking for help and advice, to sustain a good working relationship. However, I'm sure many instructors want to know from a legal standpoint what their rights are. For instance, what if the employer-employee relationship is already strained? Should any agreements be signed to protect the instructor? How should the instructor deal with existing clients who want to move to his or her new studio?

OWEN: Typically, you will work for another studio before striking out on your own. You should let your employer know your intentions but consider your employer's perspective and be mindful of the timing of that discussion. In most situations, if an employee comes to his or her current employer and advises that employer that he or she is quitting and becoming a competitor, the employer is not going to be overly eager to provide assistance. The employer will be especially concerned about the employee poaching current clientele for the new venture. Thus, if you are going to open up a studio in the same geographic region, when you advise your employer of your intentions, assume that will be your last day of work for that employer. If, however, you are opening up a studio in a different geographic region such that your employer will not be concerned about competition, your employer will be more likely to want you to continue working for a period of time and may be more helpful with some of the start-up issues you will face.

Whether you are opening a competing studio or not, it is imperative that you endeavor to maintain a good relationship since you will both, hopefully, be involved in the same industry for many years to come. However, do not take your employer's trade secrets with you—his or her client lists (even if these are clients that you worked with, they are the customers of the employer), vendor lists, etc. Remember that your employer still has his or her business to run, which will be your employer's primary focus. While you still work there, your employer will expect it to be your primary focus as well.

> **Tip:** If you signed an employment agreement, that contract will likely contain terms concerning your obligations both while you are employed and after you leave that employment. Accordingly, as part of your planning process, take some time to read over your employment agreement and, perhaps, speak with a lawyer. You will want some clear information concerning your ongoing obligations, if any, to your soon-to-be former employer.

Amy: For those people who have never seen a lawyer before, what should they expect in an initial consultation?

Owen: First, you'll want to make telephone contact with your prospective attorney and set up the initial consultation. Find out if the initial consultation is free of charge on the phone so there are no surprises when you arrive. Many attorneys will provide a free initial consultation, but do not expect a whole lot of substantive work and definitive opinions and advice if this is the case. Basically, use this opportunity to gauge whether this is someone who seems competent and who you feel comfortable working with. You will want to be prepared to lay out what it is you want to do concisely. Ideally, you will have some basic information that will assist in driving the discussion. You should have a concept of what your business ideally will look like in the first year of operation: What kind of rent can you afford? What kind of space can you get for that rent? How many employees or contractors will you need? What is a realistic number of clients to start off with? How are you going to get clients?

You will need to have money to start up your business. Do not be offended if an attorney asks you what you have for start-up costs. From the standpoint of substantive assistance, basically, your lawyer should have some clear ideas about how the business should be structured, some contacts in the community of professionals you will likely need to engage, including CPA's and commercial realtors, some ideas and opinions about what legal assistance you will need at a minimum, and what you will need as you move forward. There should be some discussion about financing. Obviously, it has to be someone you feel comfortable with, and ideally it's going to be someone who understands what you do. If you're opening a Pilates studio, it would be great if the lawyer you're working with, if nothing else, has done Pilates and understands it conceptually, or works with other businesses that have very similar setups, like a yoga studio.

Amy: What else would you recommend that a client do to prepare for an initial consultation—should the client bring any particular documents?

Owen: Other than the knowledge items discussed above, you really don't need to bring in anything. Based on my knowledge of how the Pilates world works, I would think that you have to be aligned with one of the methodologies of Pilates, whether it's STOTT® or one of the others out there, and have a clear understanding of how that works and so on. You just need to bring in your concept and show an understanding of the market. Remember, the initial interview is not only for the purpose of you sizing up the lawyer, but also for the lawyer to get a read on you. I have had many occasions where a new client comes in and, although not very well financed, he or she shows a level of enthusiasm, intelligence, and planning that indicates to me that this person has a real shot at creating a successful business. I, like anyone else, like to look at my list of clients and take particular joy in those clients who I have helped achieve significant levels of success from humble beginnings.

AMY: Would you recommend reading up on anything first? For instance, should a new client have some basic knowledge on business entities or certain types of agreements?

OWEN: It would be great to get some basic knowledge on business entities, especially corporations and limited liability companies. You can go to the Secretary of State Web site of any state and find some basic information on the entities that the state recognizes, and some basic information on how to set them up. There is no magic to setting up these entities. I think an intelligent individual can do it on his or her own, but you may want to consult with somebody to make a determination of which kind of entity you want before going there. I think the other thing that's really helpful is a basic understanding of accounting or bookkeeping principles. I don't think you have to be a tax expert or an accounting expert, but just have a basic understanding of maybe how to use QuickBooks®, and know the basic inputs that are involved and so on because that may be a significant factor. Then you're going to have to deal with the phone company and all the utility companies just like you would with any other business, and that's information you're either going to have or you're going to learn.

You need to have an understanding of marketing and you need to have a marketing plan before you open the doors. You can do everything right, but if you do not get people to walk in and put down their money for your services, you will not be successful.

Opening a Pilates studio is a very customer-service oriented business—to the extreme. When you're teaching Pilates, you are touching people and working very closely with them. You should have experience teaching Pilates, and an understanding of the boundaries and how to operate within them. It's also important to know how to manage a workforce. It may not be significant off the bat, but ideally, if you're successful it will become significant.

TIP: To find information about your state's rules and filing requirements for corporate entities, simply type "Secretary of State" and the name of your state into a search engine. Be sure that you aren't duped by the proprietary sites that have "Secretary of State" in their tags and titles; they will charge extra fees to submit corporate filings.

AMY: What else differentiates opening a Pilates studio from other business endeavors?

OWEN: This is my experience from my work with yoga studios, health clubs, and Pilates studios: essentially, the way you're going to make money is one-on-one client work. You can certainly have your mat classes, and ideally you will fill those classes and make money from them, but the real way you make money is by having someone pay you $75 or $125 an hour to do one-on-one training. In a yoga studio, for instance, you can take a much more scattershot approach to getting people to come in. They're going to pay you $15 an hour to be in this sweaty room, do a series of poses, and leave, and then you fill the room again for the next hour. For Pilates, you have to really know the demographics of the location that you're in and hone in on those who are going to be willing to pay a good sum of money for a personalized, one-on-one training experience. The people who will pay $75 to $125 an hour for a training session are usually quite different, and certainly have quite different expectations, than those who will pay $15 an hour for their towel-sized space in a room of 30 people. You need to figure out how you're going to get them in and how you're going to get referrals from those clients, as that's going to be your best source of business. In that way, it's very similar to a really high-end professional services firm. Your clientele is going to be distinguished by who's willing to pay. A lot of people, even people who make good money, will have a hard time paying people $75 an hour to do a workout. I would not necessarily say it's a tough sell, but it is a unique sell.

And then the other thing I've found is that when you're dealing with clientele like that, you're dealing with people who have very high expectations, and they can be very difficult. That just kind of comes with the territory.

AMY: Does a new studio owner have to worry about choosing a business name that no one else is using? There are certainly some standard names for Pilates studios, such as those that combine "Pilates" with "Core," "Movement," "Spine," "Balance," or "Center." And then there are the studio names that are not descriptive of Pilates at all, such as "Northstar," and names that are famous such that most people who know about Pilates would associate them only with Pilates, such as "STOTT."

OWEN: This is a very complex issue, and it's best to ask an attorney about the specific name you're going to use. Volumes have been written on the issue of trademarks and service marks and almost anything I say here briefly will be subject to numerous caveats and exceptions. However, as a general rule, if the name is merely descriptive of the product or service you are providing, you are not going to have to worry as much about using that name and infringing on the trademark rights of another because, in general, nobody can claim ownership of a descriptive term. Of course, the downside of using a descriptive term in your name is that you will not build up name recognition in your unique name over time, and you will not be able to prevent competitors from incorporating that same descriptive term into their names. On the other end of the spectrum, if the name is arbitrary or fanciful (think about the arbitrary mark "Apple" for computers, or the fanciful term "Xerox" for photocopy machines), then you may run into problems if another studio is already using a name that may be confusingly similar to it. Of course, if you secure and use an arbitrary or fanciful name, over time you will build up trademark rights in that name (even if you do not register the name, though I highly recommend registration) and you alone will be able to reap the benefits of that unique name recognition.

One way to rule potential names out is to look them up on the United States Patent and Trademark Office Web site (www.uspto.gov). You can search the trademark database, and if you see a direct hit for your name and it's used with goods or services that could be related to yours, it is probably not a good idea to use that mark. Additionally, it is a good idea to do a general Web search for the name you are considering. The Trademark Office database contains a listing of marks that have been applied for and those that have been registered, but this is not the full universe of businesses using a given mark in the marketplace. For a much more comprehensive analysis, there are companies that do full trademark availability searches in a wide range of databases and areas of the world.

If you have a trademark that is valuable to your business, you may choose to apply for federal or state registration. Federal applications tend to be more expensive to pursue than state applications, but a federal registration will give you a significantly broader scope of protection. Although it is possible to pursue these applications on your own, federal registrations tend to be especially complex and may require communication with an examining attorney from the USPTO. It is best to ask an attorney to file and prosecute trademark applications on your behalf.

TIP: To search for federal registrations and pending applications, go to www.uspto. gov and click the "Search" icon under the heading "Trademarks." Once you have submitted a query, you can click on the link to any mark to see the details of its registration, including its date of first use and the goods and services with which it is used. Get more information on trademarks by clicking the "Trademark" button at the top of your screen.

AMY: What would you recommend is a reasonable budget for attorney's fees if the studio owner is starting with $10,000 as an initial investment?

OWEN: This is going to vary widely by location. If you're in San Francisco, LA, New York, you're going to pay a lot more than you will in Alabama. That's a huge factor. I can talk about major metropolitan areas because that is what I know. Your initial budget is going to depend on the extent the individual is willing to self-help. The ballpark fees for start-up legal work will range anywhere from $3000 to $7000. It could end up being significantly less if the individual sets up her own corporation, gets her own tax ID number, and registers her own domain name. These are all things that are doable by the reasonably intelligent person, but many people are just afraid to go out and find the resources to do it on their own, or they don't know where to look.

One thing to keep in mind on the self-help issue: If you are going to do many things on your own, do not expect an attorney to sign off on the underlying work you have done. It is inherently unfair to present an attorney with a trademark application you have prepared and ask him to take a five-minute look at it and vouch for it when he was not involved in preparing it, knows nothing about the underlying search for the availability of the trademark, and knows nothing about the quality of the underlying work.

AMY: That is a good incentive for people to get advice from an attorney from the beginning rather than doing part of a task on their own. For those who choose to have an expert deal with the start-up issues, your estimate may seem high—especially for those who haven't worked with an attorney to open a business before. What is it the $3000 to $7000 going to cover?

OWEN: The first thing you're going to have your attorney do, typically, is negotiate your lease. That is one of those things you couldn't peg a hard dollar to because there's another party involved and you never really know. Then you may have an independent contractor agreement with someone who is working with you or various agreements with other suppliers that you'd have your attorney look at—everything from the copy machine to the cleaning service, things along those lines. Then you have the entity formation. Forming an entity is a relatively easy thing to do, and it's easier the fewer people involved. A one-person entity is straightforward. As soon as you have two or more people, you have to have some kind of agreement between all the individual members of that entity as to how they are going to deal with each other. So that adds a layer of complexity. There will also be some initial interaction with a CPA explaining the entity set-up, the tax ID number, and how the business is going to work. The client may already have a CPA, or any reasonable attorney should have several references. The business owner may also have an agreement with a third party that is usually going to get him or her customers or provide the system of Pilates that he or she will teach.

AMY: The new studio owner is making significant investment in these services. Are there any warning signs that people should be aware of when they enter into a new relationship with an attorney?

OWEN: Responsiveness is key. An attorney should almost always get back to you within 24 hours. Obviously, attorneys will go on vacation, but they should advise you of that ahead of time and have someone designated to get back to you if it's not him or her. There may be situations, periodically, where the attorney gets back to you in a couple days, and that's okay as long as it is not common. Related to that, you need to get the sense that your attorney is hearing you and not just talking to you. Remember, this is your business and you have your ideas that you wish to implement. Your attorney may think your ideas raise particular issues and express those concerns to you, but ultimately, it is your decision how to proceed.

Obviously, if the bills are insane, that's an issue as well. That is hard to gauge because fees and clients' needs vary so widely. But if you think that your bill is too high, certainly speak up about it.

TIP: If you're looking for the right attorney or CPA, be sure to ask your colleagues for referrals. This is a good way to find someone who is right for your business. Also, organizations like the North American Studio Alliance (www.namasta.com/1-877-NAMASTA) offer a low-cost legal referral service and low-cost distance learning on legal topics.

AMY: What would you recommend for people who want to cut costs? You've mentioned that the client can negotiate the lease, create a business entity, get a tax ID number, and register domain names. Any other tips?

Don't forget that it is possible to work for trade with an attorney. This also is related to finding an attorney who understands what you do and is interested in what you do. For instance, I was training with a client who opened a Pilates studio here in San

Francisco. I went in for a private session, stood on the Cadillac, and performed a move as instructed. I realized that if a client were to fall, he or she could really get injured. This reminded me to prepare a waiver form for my client to use with her customers.

AMY: What is it about Pilates that interests you?

OWEN: I'm interested in Pilates on a couple levels. All physical activity interests me, and all new exercise regimens and their arc of development interest me both on a physical level and from a business standpoint. I am very interested in how someone takes a routine and physical activity and builds a legal wall of protection around it, and makes money off it—which is an incredibly difficult thing to do. I think I first got interested when I saw how Spinning® was created. It still amazes me that this guy got people to buy into riding a stationary bike in a room with a bunch of other people to music for an hour and made a ton of money off of it. Just think about it—if somebody would've presented that to you at the outset, you might say it's ridiculous. But it was wildly successful and I have been spinning for years now.

AMY: And some may say there are parallels in Pilates. Having a "workout" that isn't necessarily cardiovascular, utilizes equipment that doesn't look like conventional fitness equipment, and can be focused on rehabilitation rather than just getting fit may have seemed like an impossible feat. But now millions of people have tried it and many of those people are investing in private sessions with certified instructors because the method works.

OWEN: I agree. Pilates fits into a unique niche. It is a workout but it also has a rehabilitation focus. I think Pilates and other methodologies that incorporate both the workout/fitness aspect and the rehabilitation aspect are going to be increasingly popular as the baby-boom generation ages. We now see, and increasingly will see, people in their sixties, seventies, eighties and beyond actively pursuing their fitness goals and maintaining their desire to participate in the sports and other physical activities they have participated in throughout their lives. Unlike past generations, people want to continue to participate meaningfully in physical activity as they age. This will require two things: a safe means to maintain their fitness, and a safe, personalized, and accessible means to rehabilitate from injuries that are inevitable as we age.

Personally, I get very excited when I realize that through Pilates and other fitness and rehabilitation means, I should be able to continue to play baseball, ride my bike through the Marin Headlands, and take part in serious mountain climbing right up to the day I die. It may not be fast or pretty, but I intend to do that and I am pretty certain I will need the assistance of Pilates and other regimens. And I certainly know that I am not alone in this desire. So this goes back to one of the first questions you asked in this interview—what makes a good client? A good client is someone who has something that can draw an audience. Draw a crowd of participants. I believe Pilates has the ability to draw customers and ultimately it will be up to those opening Pilates studios, teaching Pilates, and showing its benefits to broaden its reach.

> **TIP:** If your attorney understands or takes Pilates, he or she is likely to be much more aware of issues in your business than someone who has never taken a Pilates class. You also may feel more comfortable with each other from the outset because you will have that common ground. Don't forget that this also creates the potential to trade services.

Don't Forget Your Blueprint!

As Owen emphasizes, it is important to have a clear idea of how you will run your business when you meet with an attorney. It may be even more important to have a clear idea of how you'll run your business if you do to tackle some of the legal groundwork on your own. After all, you will have to be completely on top of your needs, and if you forget to address an issue that is crucial to your business, you deal with the consequences.

The worksheets in this book can help you do this! Bring them into your initial consultation if you meet with an attorney or just keep them handy for your own reference—use them to stay organized and focused. Chapter 5 will provide a budget worksheet, Chapters 8 and 9 a schedule and price list. Once you have completed each of the worksheets in this book, you will have considered both emotional/interpersonal and legal/business issues. Just by completing the worksheets, you may have answered at least some questions your attorney or CPA will ask.

The clearer an idea you have of how your business will start, grow, and become successful, the more likely you are to find people who are in tune with your goals and can help you achieve them. These people will be invaluable resources as you build the foundation for your new studio. You may even find a mentor in the process—after all, they are inspired entrepreneurs as well!

WORKSHEET: LEGAL CHECKLIST

Take this checklist with you to your initial consultation with your attorney, or use it as a task list. The "essentials" are based on the business model suggested in this book. There is plenty of space for you to fill in your own categories—your business and legal needs are as individual as you and your new studio!

Essentials

- ☐ Negotiate your lease
- ☐ Form your new business entity
- ☐ Purchase insurance
- ☐ Draft new client forms that include basic personal information and liability waivers
- ☐ ---
- ☐ ---
- ☐ ---
- ☐ ---

Extras

- ☐ Go over your current employment agreement to determine your responsibilities to your employer
- ☐ Negotiate a contract with a graphic designer
- ☐ Draft agreements regarding referrals and responsibilities with other professionals in your business network
- ☐ Negotiate an agreement with your cleaning service
- ☐ Draft agreements for your employees and independent contractors
- ☐ Apply for federal and/or state registrations of your trademarks and service marks

- ☐ Understand the warranties and service agreements on any other major office supplies you have, such as your computer, printer, or copy machine
- ☐ Understand your responsibilities with regard to your certifying organization
- ☐ Understand the warranties on your equipment
- ☐ --
- ☐ --
- ☐ --
- ☐ --
- ☐ --
- ☐ --
- ☐ --
- ☐ --

Notes:

How Much Capital Do You Really Need?

CHAPTER FIVE

HOW MUCH CAPITAL DO YOU REALLY NEED?

Answer: You can start your own Pilates studio for as little as $10,000!

Do you think I'm crazy? Did you just assume it would be more? Did you hope it would be less? I am going to show you how ten thousand bucks will give you a wonderful, personalized studio space that your clients will love.

Can you start a studio with less money? Of course you can—you just need to do it differently. I have known teachers, like my mentor Aimee McDonald, who started with a chair and six mats. Phone books wrapped in nice paper were our pillows. Ten wooden poles from Home Depot were our "small apparatus." Slowly, Aimee started building the studio and buying equipment. First she purchased some fitness circles, then flex bands, then a ball. She didn't have to buy all of the equipment at once.

A smaller investment can still turn into a successful studio. Although you may think the more money the better, more money and more equipment can lead to more problems. I have seen very expensive studios open up and fail after only a few months. The amount of money you spend upfront has very little to do with the success of your studio. Therefore, don't overspend. You don't need the burden of extra mounting invoices that you have to pay off while you are trying to start a business.

To build a successful studio, you have to start with a carefully planned budget (as with any new business), and this chapter will guide you through it.

The first question you need to ask yourself is what size you want your studio to be. For instance, if you want to manage your studio by yourself, look at spaces between 500 and 800 ft^2 in size. You can't make good use out of 1,000 square feet all by yourself, but you will need at least 400 square feet as the bare minimum. Anything in between those sizes goes! We will discuss this issue in more detail in the next chapter.

Keep in mind that it is you who runs the show, and you still have a life outside your studio. So don't rent a space that will cost you so much per month that you are working the first two weeks of a month just for the rent—you will not enjoy these two weeks, and it will be difficult to plan a vacation or days off to reward yourself for your hard work. The rent is the most important bit of overhead you have to consider. You may need up to four months to get all the technical details of your business worked out. Start small, expand slowly, and really take off later.

Try to keep your monthly rent and utility bills below $1,000—once your studio is established, aim to earn this money in less than a week per month. You'll significantly reduce your worries about this piece of overhead.

Once you have found your studio space, your focus should be on making it [your space], as you will spend most of your working hours in there with your clients. So you have to feel relaxed and balanced in the space, and at the same time offer your clients an atmosphere in which they feel relaxed as well, where they can wind down from the outside world and just focus on themselves. After all, your clients will pay you a significant amount of money per hour, and part of what they're paying for is the right environment.

Remember when I talked about caring for yourself so you can give to others at the beginning of the book? Clients sense your state of mind. Believe me, there is nothing worse than a stressed teacher in an empty studio who starts throwing out promotional offers right left and center or complaining about business. Clients will know you are desperate. Who wants to go to a desperate person, buried in debt, for balance and training? Would you?

Start small and relaxed. Leave time and energy for doing some good and pursuing your interests. The key to success is staying small and knowing when to expand. Imagine this: You will be bursting at the seams. People will want a spot in your busy schedule. Your studio will be a Pilates boutique, an impeccably run place where care and individuality are your concern. This type of studio has clients who will stay forever.

And, you will probably make about the same amount of money as any person who is driving herself crazy with a huge studio, and you will have much more free time. Which studio owner do you want to be?

Just imagine yourself for a moment with a studio that can take on five private clients at the same time. You will employ at least three other Pilates trainers and have a front desk, separate locker rooms, showers, and several restrooms. You have to invest four times the amount of money into equipment and initial renovation of the space as you would for a small studio. And your rent would be three times as high. You will get into issues such as payroll, employee benefits, human resource management, and all of the issues that come along with having several employees (short-term notice of an employee being sick, dealing with employees moving on, and so on).

Before you realize what you have gotten yourself into, you are managing a business full time rather than providing your clients with Pilates training. And you will spend a considerable amount of time managing your employees. Will you make more money with this approach? Maybe so, but will more money be worth becoming a business manager rather than a Pilates instructor? Would you accept making less money if you could keep your studio small and under your own control?

My recommendation here is to stay small and to at least start your studio by yourself. If you are able to come up with an investment of $10,000 by tapping into your savings or getting a personal loan, the budget I suggest gives you a comprehensive guide on how to spend it. If you are starting with less capital, just get rid of those items that are not crucial and adjust the amount of small equipment to fit your space.

Your $10,000.00 Pilates Studio

1. Remodeling your new Pilates studio:

Painting	$300.00
Flooring	$800.00
Lighting	$600.00
Dimmer & Fresh Outlet Plates	$100.00
Subtotal for studio renovation	$1,800.00

2. Fill your studio with some life

Mini-Refrigerator	$200.00
Stereo	$100.00
Storage	$100.00
Vaccum, electric kettle, etc.	$300.00
Subtotal for small appliances	$700.00

3. Bring on the equipment

Reformer	$2,500.00
Cadillac	$2,500.00
2 Arc Barrels	$300.00
6 Mats	$600.00
Flex bands, poles, fitness circles, foam rollers	$400.00
Boxes & other small equipment	$400.00
Subtotal for equipment	$6,700.00

4. Get the show rolling

Signage, schedules, flyers, postcards	$200.00
Business Cards	$100.00
Local advertising, basic Web site	$500.00
Subtotal for initial marketing	$800.00

Overall Startup Investment:	$10,000.00

Table caption: Most Pilates equipment these days comes from the United States, which is why I have decided to keep budgetary numbers in U.S. dollars. My experience with several studios in Europe is that you can assume a 1:1 exchange rate to the euro as this reflects the local buying power. If you deal in British pounds, just divide all figures by 1.5 for an approximate budget.

Depending on your individual situation, there might be a few other things that you have to consider in your budget. If you are going into a partnership for your Pilates space and you want to make sure that you and your partner's agreements are legally sound, you might want to add approximately $500 in attorneys' fees for a basic consultation. You might need to set up health insurance or lease a vehicle through your new business. All these things should be budgeted in from the beginning to avoid surprises later on.

There are several ways to spend less than the magic $10,000—just have a close look at the budget. For those of you who don't have $10,000, here are some tips and things to consider:

- Maybe you already own some of the small equipment pieces because you like to have them available for yourself. Obviously, you don't have to buy them again! Use what you already have.

- Another way to cut the budget down is to buy used equipment. It is also a great idea to keep your eyes and ears open for equipment manufacturer specials on exhibition pieces of equipment. Manufacturers don't want to ship the pieces they had on display at a show back to their warehouses, and they are willing to give big discounts as long as you get your own transportation for the equipment.

- Depending on your education and your certifying organization, you might be eligible for manufacturer discounts. Ask the manufacturers for discounts and get quotes from different companies. Call back and negotiate. Usually, you can talk your way into a 20 – 25% discount if you are persistent.

Equipment: What to buy?

Once you are certified, the temptation begins. You have the education—now you want the stuff. Do you really need all of it? If your space allows for it, I would start with a Reformer, mats, and small apparatus. Then add a Cadillac or consider buying a Reformer/Trapeze combination unit. Adding some barrels and exercise balls will give you plenty of flexibility to make workouts creative and challenging.

What about the Chair and Ladder Barrel? In all honesty, I would suggest you hold off on those. For most clients who you will see once or twice per week, the chair is not a great option. After all, in those two hours, we are trying desperately to get them out of those patterns they are already in. Sitting would just reinforce what we are trying to balance. You need a fairly advanced or very regular client (three times per week minimum) to make the Chair a valuable investment. The long-standing myth that the

HOW MUCH CAPITAL DO YOU REALLY NEED?

Chair is supposed to be great for pregnant women is rebutted by Carolyne Anthony, a prenatal/postpartum education expert: "I don't think that it is particularly indicated during pregnancy. There are gentler ways, for example using the exercise ball."

As for the Ladder Barrel, I would also hold off on purchasing that. In my experience, few clients, aside from dancers, can balance on that thing and do abdominal exercises. I would hold back on purchasing this piece of equipment until you really have a strong demand for it, unless you teach your city's ballet troupe...

Lynette Rasmussen, a physical therapist at the University of Michigan Spine Program, has a totally different thought on the Ladder Barrel. She says, "I am a physical therapist and not a dancer, and yet I love the Ladder Barrel. I use it even with advanced beginner clients who also seem to like it."

My point is to choose your equipment wisely, depending on your budget. This will be a personal choice, and it will depend on your needs as well as the needs of your clients. For the first year, you will be perfectly happy with fewer pieces of equipment. Then add on later.

I've mentioned some ways to cut equipment costs, but one thing you should not compromise on is the quality of equipment you buy. A $700 Reformer bought over the Internet or from a television infomercial is neither safe nor long lasting. These pieces of equipment are designed to soothe people's bad consciences and be a substitute for actually exercising more often, and they will soon end up in the closet next to some other piece of abandoned fitness equipment. Your studio needs professional equipment that is designed to be used many hours per day over several years. Only a professional Reformer will hold up under this fatigue. After approximately four years, you will need to replace bits and pieces of a solid Reformer for the first time (e.g., the rollers). Until then, a professional Reformer is virtually maintenance free and just needs good cleaning. Be smart about buying your equipment!

Another way to reduce your initial budget is to cut remodeling costs. Maybe you found a place with a good wooden floor that needs some care. If your husband, wife, significant other, best friend, brother-in-law, or whoever you engage to do your studio remodeling is a DIY expert, you can actually save quite a bit of money. It will be the pride of whoever helps you to come up with smart and cost-effective solutions.

Ask around in your network of friends—maybe someone still has an old refrigerator around that you can "borrow." Even if it's unsightly, just hide its 70's design behind a curtain; your clients can enjoy a crisp bottle of water without seeing the refrigerator itself! Maybe someone has a second vacuum cleaner that you can have, or there might be a boom box at your house that isn't used. Get started with these, and you can always upgrade later.

So, you can start your own Pilates studio with as little as $5,000, and you don't have to compromise on quality or be satisfied with something that looks cheap.

There are some important things to keep in mind during the start-up phase of your new studio.

1. Keep your old job unless it is in another private studio.

Obviously, your studio will not start out fully booked; it has to grow, and you have to grow with it. Even though I've explained how this growth will happen over the first few months, it might be a good idea to keep your current job part time as a leg to stand on. Unfortunately, this is not an option if you are already working in a private Pilates studio that might be a competitor to your studio. Make sure there is no conflict of interests.

If there is no conflict because your current job has nothing to do with private Pilates classes, use your current job to meet people and tell them about your new endeavors—always have a business card and a postcard or flyer ready!

2. Fight for discounts.

No matter how much money you spend initially on your studio equipment, it will probably end up being the lion's share of your overall spending. You might be eligible for some discounts on equipment if you buy it through your certifying organization, but you will have to ask!

Before you start making calls to order equipment, it is a good idea to know the market. What other companies offer the equipment you need? What are their list prices? Be sure to figure out the price with tax and delivery to your studio—you'll be surprised how much difference the shipping policies of equipment manufactures can make. How much equipment can you buy in a bundle to gain a better position for negotiation?

Once you know all the facts, you should obtain quotes from various manufacturers and distributors. Now it is time to call the sales person who gave you the quote and ask for a better price, a higher discount, free shipping, etc. If you don't feel up for talking to a well-trained sales rep, use email. You can probably save between 10% and 20% through some negotiating, which can add up to hundreds of dollars overall. The first response you get is never the bottom line—go back and ask for more!

Your rule of thumb should be: If I spend more than $5,000 on equipment at one place, I deserve at least a 25% discount.

Use the following checklist as a guide:

- ✓ What piece(s) of equipment do I need to purchase?

- ✓ Create a table that includes all manufacturers and distributors, individual list prices, taxes, and shipping costs.

- ✓ Get quotes in writing.

- ✓ Contact manufacturers, distributors, and your certifying organization for discounts.

- ✓ Negotiate.

3. Purchase insurance on day one.

Yes—we all hate buying insurance. It always makes us feel like we are paying too much money for not enough support. Remember that you are about to start a business in which you have close contact with people. You will touch clients, and they are performing physically demanding exercise under your supervision on equipment that is heavy and can be hazardous. You will be taking on some responsibility for their safety.

The risk of injuring someone in your studio may be unlikely if you are well educated in teaching Pilates and have sufficient expertise and apprenticeship (we are talking more than 1,000 hours). But if your client gets injured, it may be very difficult to prove that it wasn't your fault. Although having a liability disclaimer that your clients sign when you start to work together is good practice, it will not prevent possible liability claims.

There are several organizations, including NAMASTA, that offer insurance for Pilates instructors and studio owners. The policies are often more affordable if you are a member of an association that negotiates group rates with insurance companies. These associations also require that you are a certified trainer, as that obviously limits their risk. Contact information for NAMASTA is in the additional resources section at the end of this book.

Once you've purchased insurance coverage, there is no need to stress about these issues. In our experience of running small Pilates studios over the past six years, we did not have a single case of injury that was caused by or accused of happening through Pilates training. The best way to protect yourself is to take notes after each class you had with a client. Document comments your clients made, which exercises you performed, and what the immediate feedback was. Good documentation may very well help you create a strong case for yourself in the event of a claim against you.

4. Keep your studio clean and tidy.

From the first day your studio opens, it should be the cleanest place in town. Private clients will come to you to relax, exercise, and get away from their busy days in the outside world—they want to feel completely comfortable. They deserve a pristine environment. However, these clients themselves will bring dust and dirt into the studio no matter what season it is, and they will make the mats and equipment dirty. Sooner or later you might see eight clients per day, and your beautiful studio will be filthy...

Unless you love cleaning more than anything else (if so, give us a call!), you should outsource this burden from day one. In the beginning, when you are not fully booked, you might get away with a professional coming in once a week to clean your studio thoroughly. But you still have to vacuum the floors and clean every surface in the bathroom in between professional cleanings, and wipe off all equipment after it is used. As soon as you are booking more clients, you should have the cleaning done twice per week.

Yes, this will eventually add about $50 per week to your overhead. Even though cleaning may not be something you hear successful studio owners talking about, it will be an important part of your business that will keep clients coming back.

Please make sure that whoever you hire to clean your studio does not use any products containing bleach. You don't want your studio to smell like a hospital. A mild citrus cleaner will do a better job for you. Lynette Rasmussen suggests a couple of drops of Dr. Bronner's organic soap added to essential oils for a great smelling cleanser. You want the place to feel clean, not antiseptic!

This may sound like a lot of things you have to consider, and $10,000 is certainly no small amount of money, but once you set your mind on it you will find out how much fun it is to get started. You are creating something totally new and have the opportunity to design it the way you want and that expresses yourself. You are the one in charge, and you deserve all the credit for it. It will take a few months to a year to get from the idea of having your own Pilates space to the grand opening. You will have to find time during that period for all the little things that have to be kept in mind and have to be organized—do it at your own pace.

Notes:

1. Remodeling your new Pilates studio:

Painting	$
Flooring	$
Lighting	$
Dimmer + outlet plates	$
Subtotal	$

2. Fill your studio with some life:

Mini-refrigerator	$
Stereo	$
Shelving	$
Other appliances, etc.	$
Subtotal	$

3. Bring on the equipment:

Reformer	$
Cadillac	$
Wunda Chair	$
Ladder Barrel	$
Arc Barrels	$
Mats	$
Flex bands, poles, foam rollers, fitness circles	$
Boxes and other small equipment	$
Subtotal	$

4. Get the show rolling:

Sinage	$
Schedules	$
Postcards	$
Business cards	$
Local advertising	$
Basic Web site	$
Subtotal	$

Totals:

1. Remodeling	$
2. Furniture	$
3. Equipment	$
4. Marketing	$
Total Startup Investment	$

Notes:

Location, Location, Location!

CHAPTER SIX

Neighborhood

As with any location decisions, the market analysis has to come first. You need to determine whether there is a market for a Pilates studio where you want to open one. If there are already studios in that area, it is a good indication that a market is established. However, once you know there is a market, you have to consider whether another studio could thrive alongside the others.

If the city where you are opening your studio is big (over 250,000 people), you shouldn't be concerned about a few other studios in the area. However, if you want to open a studio in a smaller town, you have to investigate whether there is a market for a Pilates studio that offers private sessions. It is possible that all the potential clients are happy with the low-key offerings of their local gym.

You are about to offer a service that is primarily for private clients at a price of $50 to $95 per hour, so the neighborhood where your studio is located needs to reflect this fact. Opening a studio in an area where everyone is destitute probably will not work. Opening it in a strip mall on the edge of town will make it hard to attract the right clientele.

Your private clients will come to your studio for one or two sessions per week. Everyone has a tight schedule these days, and no one likes to spend time finding a parking space. Ideally, your studio will offer parking or be located less than a block away from a public parking structure. If you are lucky enough to live in an area that offers public transportation, your studio's distance from the next station will make a big difference in its success.

As a guideline, just think about what makes you feel comfortable when you go to a place that provides you with personal treatment and what turns you off.

Competition Analysis

Obviously, the idea of opening a Pilates studio is not brand new. In a lot of areas, there are already several studios established. This does not necessarily mean that there isn't enough business out there for your studio as well, but you have to look at the competition carefully before setting up shop.

Studios in the same city often start competing rather than working together, even if collaborating would make life easier for everyone. You don't want to open your studio right across the street from an existing studio, not so much because you would impose on the existing business, but more because it is unlikely you would take clients from a studio that is well established.

It is a good idea to check out all Pilates studios that cater to the nearest 250,000 people. In a metropolitan city, you may only cover one quarter of that city. In a small town, you may visit all the studios in the whole city plus those in the outskirts and surrounding townships. Go and set up appointments with each studio and take a few classes. Be sure to visit the gyms that offer Pilates as well as the Pilates-only studios. Make notes of what you like and dislike, what clientele frequents the studio, whether the studio has waiting lists (a good sign that it is successful and that there is more market potential), how experienced and well educated the teachers are, and which organization certified those instructors. Use a chart to organize your notes, including sections such as:

Competitor's Space	Studio Staff	Marketing
Atmosphere	Trainer knowledge	Web site
Parking	Frendliness of staff	Pricing
Location	Method of training	Policies
Lighting	Equipment	
Cleanness		
Facilities		

Pricing is very important, as it will provide you with a good feel for the average rates for private and group classes in your particular area.

Rate each aspect immediately after leaving the studio, and write down any distinctive comments that come to mind.

Once you have visited each studio and go back over your notes, you will be amazed at how much useful information and how many new ideas you will have for your own studio. For each of your categories, find the best studio in that category. This becomes the benchmark that you set for your own studio!

LOCATION, LOCATION, LOCATION!

Next, locate all the other studios in your area on a map and find an empty spot that still meets all your other criteria. This is the area where you want to look for the appropriate space, keeping the Location Checklist at the end of this chapter handy. You are looking for a space that has these features:

- Attracts the right clientele

- Good neighborhood

- Next studio far enough away

- Easy to find

- Parking available and/or close to public transportation

If you feel comfortable in the studios that you visit, you might as well be honest and talk to the studio owners about your intentions to open your own place. There is only one thing that is absolutely off limits: approaching that studio's clients and talking to them about your plans to open another studio. This would be the fastest way to lose all the support in your community. You will need support down the road for organizing workshops with other studios, finding substitutes for when you are on vacation, or attending conferences. You will be happier when you get along with the other Pilates teachers in town. You are bound to run into them sooner or later at social events or in your daily life, and that will be much more comfortable if you have a good rapport with them.

Getting along with other Pilates instructors in your community is even more important if you are already working as a teacher in one of the studios in town. In that case, you probably know better than anyone else about that studio's strengths and weaknesses. You are already in a difficult situation because you are about to leave that studio to become a competitor.

Be open, honest, and a team player! Involve the studio owner who has employed you in your plans of opening your own studio. Prepare for this meeting well, as your success as a studio owner will depend on how this meeting goes. Obviously, no one at your current studio will be excited about the news of more competition, especially from their own coworker. Therefore, it is very important to keep a few dos and don'ts in mind:

- Be very clear that you will not take any clients with you. (There are legal strings attached to this, and it is strongly recommended to seek advice from a lawyer if you do have current clients who plan to move to your new studio.)

- Make sure that your studio will be a sufficient distance away from the place that employed you.

- Point out the differences between your own studio and the one you are leaving.

- Don't even think about trying to employ trainers of the current studio at yours, even though they are friends. It will always look like you are stealing resources, no matter how good your intentions may be.

- Offer an informal partnership and continuing teamwork. Help each other by substituting for each other, trading clients with special needs, etc.

If everything goes well, you will have laid the foundation for a strong network between your current studio and your new business.

Size Matters!

In Chapter 5, I discussed the issue of size from a budgeting point of view. I discussed the impact the size of a space has on your monthly overhead. You must be able to support the monthly lease on your own without putting a burden on yourself that will cause sleepless nights. After all, this kind of business should be fun!

Now, let's talk about size from the perspective of finding the right space for your studio. Keep in mind that you don't need a huge space for several large pieces of equipment. When working with private clients, you can only use one piece of equipment at a time. As far as big equipment is concerned, you don't need much more than a Reformer and maybe a Cadillac. If you want to provide small mat classes at your studio, you need space for five mats to fit comfortably. One large room should do it, but an extra small room can be very valuable for expanded offerings like massage or Gyrotonic®, or even to rent out to another Pilates teacher.

As you may recall from Chapter 5, a Pilates studio that is managed by one person should be between 500 and 800 ft². It should include one to two rooms plus a bathroom (or access to a common bathroom), and if possible, a kitchenette. If you are planning to open your Pilates space with a partner (see Chapters 3 and 4), you might need a little more room. But keep in mind that if you work with a partner, it is best to choose a space that one of you could manage on your own if necessary. What if your partner leaves for an extended vacation or intensive training for a few months? What if your partner is ill and cannot teach? What if your partnership does not work out? It is best to be prepared. Also, each one of you will only work a certain number of hours per week (30 hours at the most). With some creative scheduling, you and your partner should be able to use a smaller space efficiently rather than increase the square footage.

In general there are two different kinds of leases available—commercial leases and residential leases. The residential leases are usually easier to understand and run for one year only. There is a certain vulnerability involved with this kind of lease as you might face a steep increase in rent after the first year. It is even possible that the space might not be available to you after the first year. On the other hand, your commitment is limited with a residential lease, and in case you have to move on after a year, you won't need to get out of a multi-year contract.

If you decide to enter into a commercial lease, we recommend that you seek advice from an expert who has dealt with these kinds of contracts before. Commercial leases include a lot of fine print that is generally difficult to interpret. If you are acting as a sole proprietor, you may not want to enter into this kind of lease. See Chapter 4 for more information.

Once you find the perfect space that is the right size, you have to research pricing for such a space in the area. Unless you are in the heart of Manhattan or San Francisco, you do not want to spend more than $800 to $1,000 for a monthly lease, as this seems to be the threshold amount for high stress and sleepless nights. I saw one case in which a studio owner spent over $3,000 per month for 2,000 ft^2 in a strip mall at the edge of town. The business failed after only a few months.

Your ideal studio is:

- 500 to 800 square feet

- Less than $1,000 monthly lease

If either the square footage or the price of a potential space doesn't fit, let it go. Don't start your new business with a compromise!

Notes:

WORKSHEET: LOCATION CHECKLIST

Take some notes on each location you visit and then check the box
for each criterion that space fulfills.

Addresses

1. _____

2. _____

3. _____

4. _____

5. _____

	1	2	3	4	5
Attracts the right clientele	☐	☐	☐	☐	☐
Good neighborhood	☐	☐	☐	☐	☐
Next studio far enough away	☐	☐	☐	☐	☐
Easy to find	☐	☐	☐	☐	☐
Parking/public transportation	☐	☐	☐	☐	☐
500 – 800 ft^2	☐	☐	☐	☐	☐
Less then $1,000 monthly lease	☐	☐	☐	☐	☐

Making the
Most of Your Space

CHAPTER SEVEN

Rooms

What type of training do you want to offer in your studio space? This is what your studio layout should be based on. Your Pilates space is defined by several key factors. First, make sure the size of your space fits your needs, as discussed in Chapters 5 and 6. Second, you need to have space for at least two large pieces of equipment, possibly a Reformer and a Cadillac, with enough space around them to assist your clients. It is popular for well-established small studios to have a second Reformer and teach semi-privates. Keep this in mind and mentally reserve room for a second Reformer.

You also want to make sure that you have space for five mats to allow you to teach group classes. Keep in mind that if you offer mat classes and run them even if they are not fully booked, they can be a great marketing tool to find clients who want to excel and will book private sessions with you. There are a couple of full-size studio Reformers out there that come with wheels on one side so that they can be lifted on the opposite side and then rolled out of the way. This is a very practical feature, but don't plan on moving the equipment every day, as a good studio Reformer is heavy!

You also will appreciate a second, smaller room that you don't really need to use right away. This is the space that might start out as a changing room but might very soon be transformed into a second teaching or treatment room. Keep in mind, however, that you are not opening a big gym, so an extra changing room is not totally necessary. A nice screen will do the job and keeps your space highly flexible.

Bathroom

You need a small bathroom inside or adjacent to your studio. It should be state of the art and meticulously clean at all times. Although this may seem obvious, I have seen many places with outdated, filthy bathrooms.

Whether or not you need a shower is really up to you. Even though I have rarely had clients who actually made use of the shower in my studio, the offering itself makes a difference as to how the quality of a studio is perceived.

Windows

It is very important when looking for the right studio space to find sources of natural light and fresh air. The absolute dream space would have natural overhead light, but that is hard to find. If you can't find skylights, look for a place with plenty of windows.

Avoid a space with windows that look out onto an unkempt backyard or the wall of an adjacent building, or directly onto the street. A worst-case scenario would be a storefront where people passing by can look inside. So in most cases, the ideal studio space is above ground level with lots of natural light but no potential distractions in direct view.

As I discussed in *Survival Skills for Pilates Teachers*, natural lighting has several health benefits as well. It is one of the main sources of Vitamin D, which prevents osteoporosis. Health and is always worth the investment.

Lighting

There is nothing that comes close to natural light in creating a good atmosphere, which is very important for a Pilates studio as a place to do mind-body work. Even if you are lucky enough to find a studio with skylights, not all of your classes will happen during bright daylight, so therefore finding the right light for your studio is essential. Stay far away from fluorescent light or any other form of industrial overhead light. This sort of light might be okay for industrial work, but it is certainly not ideal for any kind of office work, much less a Pilates studio. The reason why so many offices have fluorescent lighting is because it is cheap, not because it is good for people.

Lynette Rasmussen, physical therapist at the University of Michigan Spine Program, had a lot to say about the importance of lighting. "I believe that working in fluorescent lighting is absolutely taboo. Natural lighting from the outside is crucial to an instructor. The clients come and go, no big deal, but if you are in a room with no natural lighting it can be very depressing. If you plan on hiring other instructors, you could lose them on this factor alone."

When you do need artificial lighting, you want to work with several sources of indirect light—standing lamps that direct light toward the ceiling (torch lamps, for example) provide this sort of light when they are carefully placed around the studio. Remember to make sure that there are enough electrical outlets; you don't want to clutter the studio with extension cords. This sort of indirect light in combination with a good halogen light system under the ceiling will do the trick if you make sure that each source of light can be dimmed. Halogen light provides very "clean" light without creating an atmosphere that is sterile. It is especially effective if it is used indirectly to illuminate walls, ceilings, or pictures.

Floors

When it comes to flooring in a Pilates studio, your choices are very limited. Any form of carpet should be avoided as it will be filthy after a short period of time regardless of how clean you might keep it. Any form of tiling or even concrete is out as well, as it is too hard and will always feel cold even if you install a floor heating system.

My highest recommendation goes to natural wooden floors—they are soft, warm, and very easy to clean. Unfortunately, it is not very cheap to put them into a space, and doing so is only worth it if you are going to stay in the same space for several years. If the space you found meets all other criteria except the right floor, you can still come fairly close to a wooden floor by using a laminate that is almost as good as wooden floor but a lot cheaper. Be sure to check to see if there is old hardwood flooring under the carpet in any space you are considering. If there is, bingo! Make your DIY expert or closest friends and family sweat for a weekend: Rip out the old stuff, sand the floor down, and apply a fresh coat of varnish. The hard work will pay off!

Walls

The walls in your studio need to be as straight and clutter-free as possible. A clean plastered or dry-walled studio is preferable to any kind of textured surface. No matter what has been in that space before, make it a point to give your studio a fresh coat of paint. It is best to stay away from a pure white paint as it will make your studio look like a doctor's office. Also, avoid beige or cream. These colors are for rental apartments, and they will only express a lack of creativity and character.

Take time to find your own color, and use the lightest version of that color to keep lots of light and a friendly atmosphere in your studio. Stay away from dark colors such as aubergine or bright colors such as pure red, as these colors do not make people calm down and relax. Any form of blue tends to cool rooms down, so it is best to stay away from blues unless your studio is located in an area that has very high temperatures year round. Very light yellow, fresh light orange, lime green, and warm peach are good colors that will encourage your clients to feel calm and centered yet energized and awake. Stay as pure as possible with your color choice and seek out natural, soft colors that can be associated with nature and fruit. Don't use more than two different colors in your studio. If this seems like it will be a major task, keep in mind that repainting a small studio can be done in one weekend.

Make sure that the painting is done with great care; your clients will spend hours looking at your walls and ceiling, and they will notice a sloppy paint job.

Once you have the walls freshly painted in the color that represents you and also

Pilates Space

---

offers a warm and welcoming environment to your clients, don't ruin your work by cluttering these beautiful walls with random pictures, nick-knacks, or, worst of all, motivational posters. Some of the bigger Pilates certifying organizations offer well-designed overview charts that list exercises. If you really like some of these charts, it is okay to hang them in your studio. Keep in mind that less is more!

Practical Space

Your studio should also have some extra space for your practical needs in running the business and maintaining the space.

Your studio does not have to have a separate kitchenette, but it is nice to provide tea and water to your clients. Everyone appreciates a cup of herbal tea or an individual bottle of water. This is a simple, $0.50 treat for your clients that makes them feel cared for.

At the very least, you do need a hidden corner for practical equipment and appliances: cleaning supplies, a small refrigerator, an extra fan for hot days, a small stereo system, and all the other little things that are necessary to keep your studio clean and comfortable. It is also important to make space for a desk, even if it is very small, where you can do paperwork comfortably. Even a shelf at the right height will work just fine.

When you are out there hunting for the perfect studio space, don't get overwhelmed with all the details! Use the checklist at the end of the chapter as a guide to make sure you don't overlook anything. It is a good idea to create your own checklist and personalize it with those items of your own that are important to you. Go back to the notes you took when you checked out all of the competitors' studios. It is perfectly okay to adapt some of those ideas or features to fit your own space.

WORKSHEET: STUDIO LAYOUT

This checklist for your studio layout is meant as a guideline only. Pick what you need and add what you don't want to miss.

Addresses

1. _____

2. _____

3. _____

4. _____

5. _____

Essentials	1	2	3	4	5
Space for two pieces of large equipment	☐	☐	☐	☐	☐
Space for five mats	☐	☐	☐	☐	☐
One separate room for extras	☐	☐	☐	☐	☐
Bathroom (plus a changing room or shower)	☐	☐	☐	☐	☐
_____	☐	☐	☐	☐	☐
_____	☐	☐	☐	☐	☐
_____	☐	☐	☐	☐	☐

Features	1	2	3	4	5
Windows	☐	☐	☐	☐	☐
Lighting	☐	☐	☐	☐	☐
Floors	☐	☐	☐	☐	☐
Walls	☐	☐	☐	☐	☐
Practical space (kitchenette/ space for desk)	☐	☐	☐	☐	☐
	☐	☐	☐	☐	☐
	☐	☐	☐	☐	☐
	☐	☐	☐	☐	☐
	☐	☐	☐	☐	☐
	☐	☐	☐	☐	☐

WORKSHEET: STUDIO LAYOUT

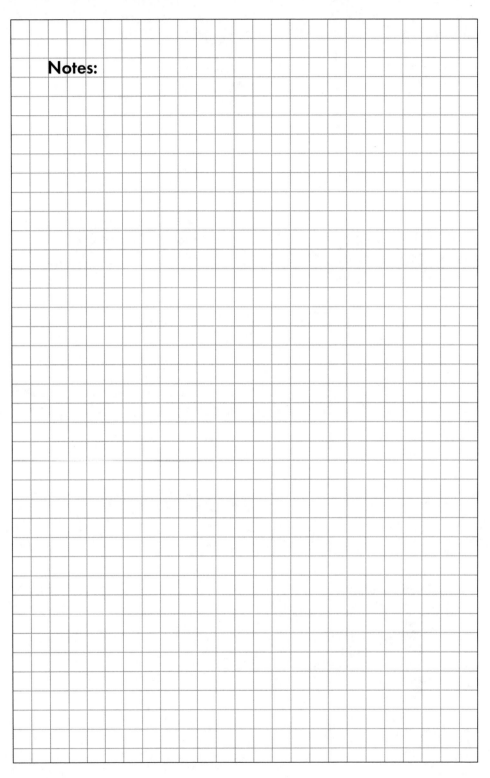

Notes:

Developing a Pricing Strategy

CHAPTER EIGHT

DEVELOPING A PRICING STRATEGY

Before getting into detail about the pricing structure of your classes, let's develop a monthly budget for your new business. We have already gone over a budget for initial expenses. This budget will help you figure out how much overhead you have to cover each month and how much you want (or need) to get out of the time you invest.

As I mentioned in Chapter 5, you want to commit to a maximum rent of $800 to $1000 per month to avoid unnecessary stress. A conservative estimate is that you will spend another $200 per month in phone bills, $200 on extras for your clients (water, granola bars, essential oils, candles, taking steady clients for lunch, etc.), and $100 on office supplies. As a rule of thumb, you should put another $100 per month aside as depreciation of your Pilates equipment plus an additional $200 per month for your continuing education (conferences, training, certifications, and travel).

There are also considerations that will vary significantly from person to person. Do you pay for your health insurance? Do you have car payments? These two expenses can quickly add up to another $700 per month depending on your individual situation. For the sample budget here, I'll leave the car and the health insurance out. However, please account for these costs in your budget if you will need to pay for them.

According to our conservative estimates, your base overhead is approximately $1,600 per month—already quite a bit of money! This amounts to $19,200 per year. So, you have $19,200 that you need to earn before a single dollar goes to you!

Monthly Studio Overhead

1. Studio rent	$800.00
2. Phone	$200.00
3. Client extras	$200.00
4. Office supplies	$100.00
5. Depreciation of equipment	$100.00
6. Continuing education	$200.00
7. Car/transportation	?
8. Health insurance	?
Total monthly overhead:	$1600.00
Annual cost of running your studio:	$19,200.00

I'm assuming that you will work 40 weeks per year. The remaining weeks will be free for you to attend conferences, go for additional training, spend time with your family and friends, and enjoy your life—after all, Pilates teachers don't have to participate in the 50-week-per-year, 40-hour-per-week corporate world. So, you need to make approximately $480 per week just to keep your studio going. This may sound like a lot, but you will be surprised at how reasonable it is. Now that we have accounted for the overhead, how much profit do you want to make?

Assuming that you will actually work in your studio 40 weeks per year, and considering the type of work you do, you should work 30 hours per week at the maximum. Keep in mind that you will have to give 100% of your energy and attention during all sessions with clients; you are working with individuals who expect your full attention to their issues and their health. Opening your studio and actually booking 30 hours a week will take about a year, so don't get impatient in the first few months of business if you still have some free hours.

For further calculations and estimates, let's assume that you will end up working 25 hours per week with clients—scheduling, organization, and accounting not included. The minimum hourly rate in the Pilates community is around $50 and the maximum tends to be around $95. What you should charge depends on several factors, including:

- How much experience you offer to your clients

- How much other studios in your area charge

- Where you want to position yourself and your studio in the marketplace

Based on the rate of $50 per class and an average working week of 25 classes, you are making $1,250 per week. After you deduct the $480 overhead estimated in the budget above, you are going home with $770 per week of taxable income. In 40 working weeks doing this "part-time" job, you are making $30,800 per year and having a lot of fun!

This income should be your baseline. You can do the math yourself: Suppose that you are able to charge $60 per class due to your experience, the average price of classes in your area, and your position in the local Pilates market. Suppose you can pump your hours up to 30 per week. You end up with over $50,000 of taxable income at the end of the year, and you still have 12 weeks of vacation time!

This all is certainly a very business-like approach to the pricing of your studio and might not be the way you like to think about pricing your classes. As an alternative, you might want consider the common approach to budgets for private studios: how much you can afford based on how much you want to work. This approach is especially good for future studio owners who already have a packed schedule due to family obligations, other jobs, or study.

The rule of thumb for this method of analysis is to figure out how much time you want to work as a Pilates studio owner and how much money you should spend on rent and other overhead based on that. Here is a golden rule that you should follow once you have been in business for two years. This rule is backed up with experience!

You should earn your monthly studio rent in three full days of work.

If you work 18 hours per week as a Pilates teacher in your own studio, this means you work approximately 11 hours in three days—which should cover the rent for the whole month. If you charge $50 per hour, you can spend $550 on your rent. Don't worry at this point about the other overhead expenses; we are only determining your initial cost structure here.

If you work 30 hours per week (basically full time) and charge $50 per hour, you will make $900 in three work days. If that is the case, you can afford a studio that is $900 per month.

How much studio can I afford?			
Hours you work per week	**Hours you work in 3 days**	**Hourly base rate**	**Maximum monthly rent**
18	11.0	$50.00	$550.00
25	15.0	$50.00	$750.00
30	18.0	$50.00	$900.00

Now that you have an idea of what your overhead will be and how much rent you can afford, let's talk a little bit about your pricing strategy.

Pricing Classes

There are four main pricing categories for classes that you may offer in your studio:

- Privates

- Mat classes

- Semi-privates

- Class cards

The most difficult task is to determine a price structure that serves your needs, attributes the right value to your abilities and your time, is acceptable in your location, and can be maintained for at least a year. Raising prices is one of the most difficult tasks for any business to do, and you want to wait to do it as long as possible after you open your studio. If you are a well-educated trainer with at least 1,000 hours of apprenticeship, you have a good reputation, and you teach in an area that has a market for Pilates training but few or no studios, you should price yourself at the higher end of the spectrum. Not everyone will be able to afford you and your time, but you will be very satisfied with your reimbursement, you will work fewer hours for the same money you would've made working more, and your satisfaction with your job will show in your work with your clients.

Be prepared to offer incentives and discounts, but only in trade for something, such as getting paid up front for a number of appointments. I'll say more on this when we get to class cards.

Private Classes

This form of Pilates training is the most common in serious Pilates studios and offers the most benefit to your clients, as they will get all of your attention. You will focus on your clients' specific needs, tend to their health issues (and possibly their private thoughts), and provide an exclusive atmosphere. All of these factors contribute to the price for a private appointment, and the exclusivity and individual attention are worth at least as much as the Pilates training itself.

These private classes should be your top-of-the-line offering. If you have some experience and a good space, a good reference point is $50 per class. But if you feel that you can charge more because your studio is in a very posh area, you should start at a higher rate.

Don't offer "introductory rates"; you are not a fitness studio that needs to gain market share quickly. On the other hand, it is a very common and fair practice to provide the first class for free so that both you and your new client can determine whether you get along and want to work with each other.

Make sure your clients pay you every time they come and see you. This reinforces the good practice of keeping their balances up to date. Also, schedule the next appointment at the end of each class; try to find out what times work best for each client and offer to book them into those spots for several weeks in advance to guarantee them a standing spot in your schedule.

Keep records of your clients' habits and their body issues. Also, keep track of their birthdays, their spouses' names, information about their children, etc. Don't forget to pamper your private clients with fresh tea, a bottle of water, a high-quality granola bar, or a piece of fruit. Your private clients will be the foundation of your business; if you treat them well, they will stay with you for a long time and stay loyal even if you cannot accommodate their time every week because you travel to conferences and take extended vacations.

Mat Classes

Mat classes are the "one-size-fits-all super combo"—everyone tries to offer them, but they rarely make good money, considering the scheduling effort that goes into them. Many studios offer them to create traffic and to fill the space that they rented. It may be best to avoid offering open mat classes to which clients can drop in without prior scheduling—the class will either be empty or overflowing, and neither situation is good. You will not have any planning security. Drop-in clients usually don't work well for a small space. You need to know who is coming and when. If people want to try a class, have them register with you ahead of time.

If you design mat classes properly, they can become a very effective marketing tool for your studio. A series of mat classes usually runs for ten weeks. As a bonus, you can offer an eleventh week as a make-up in case any students missed one of the sessions. If you manage to get a group of four or five clients together who book a series of mat classes with you, they will get to know each other during the course of the series. Before the term ends, offer your clients a consecutive class term at the next level of advancement. Keep this offering open only to those clients for a week or two so that they can take a space in the class if they want it. If your clients enjoyed the first mat class term, they will very likely book the next term right away. This offers you the advantages of upfront payments, a stable schedule, and clients you already know.

After the second term, you may find that some of your clients will want to try the equipment as well—train them on the Reformer for 30 minutes free of charge. Provide your full attention and the atmosphere you offer any of your private clients, and you might have won yourself a new private client. That client might see you once per week in the mat class and once per week individually.

If you decide to rent a small studio, your mat class should host four or five clients. They each need to sign up for one full series and pay upfront; there should be no reimbursement if they miss a class. After all, you are committing your time and studio space to them independently of whether they show up or not.

The standard price for a mat class is $15, so for a ten-week series, this adds up to $150 to be paid at the first class. If you fill the class with four people, you technically walk away with $60 per class (the same as with a private client), but your administration and scheduling in preparation for a mat class takes more time than for a standing private.

Getting the first mat class going is more difficult than you may think—you have to find the clients for it, contact them, and then offer the class. Once the class gets going and everyone enjoys it, word will spread and the clients from your first mat class will bring in more potential clients.

Semi-Privates

This form of class is usually offered for two reasons: a studio has extra pieces of certain equipment and wants to utilize them, or clients want to share their Pilates experiences with a friend, either for fun or to split the cost.

Obviously, you can only offer a semi-private class on the Reformer if you have two Reformers. Two mats aren't really enough for a semi-private, as this would be only slightly different from a mat class. A Reformer plus a Cadillac does not work either, because you can't focus on two different pieces of equipment at the same time and still protect your clients' safety. There are studios that offer semi-privates on different equipment. I was almost injured in a semi-private class in which I was working on the Reformer and the instructor was focusing on my partner's work on the Cadillac. Utilizing a different piece of equipment for each client can be dangerous.

Your goal should be to have your clients organize semi-privates. This means that clients who want semi-privates should bring the second person in, simply because it saves you the headache of finding and scheduling this second client. You will also know that the two clients get along with each other.

Schedule a semi-private the same way you would schedule a private class: Offer only the total price for both clients together, and let them do the math of splitting up the cost. Because your concentration has to be even sharper than with a single client, the price for a semi-private is higher than for a private class. You should charge at least $10 more per hour for a semi-private than for a single client. This is still a good deal for your clients, as they get to use equipment under your supervision for around $35 each. They might even think that taking a class with a friend is better than doing it on their own.

Class Cards

Class cards are a nice way to offer your clients a discount without making it look cheap. They also provide you with the huge advantage of low-effort administration and no money juggling. Here is how it works: Once you have established a good relationship with your private clients, offer them a card that contains eight to ten private classes to be paid for up front at a discount of $10 to $15 per class. If your standard rate is $60 per hour for a private class, you can offer eight classes for $400 or ten classes for $500. Your clients will certainly see the advantage in significant savings, but you benefit by getting paid upfront and having less administrative work to do. You only have to deal with a check one time, and you can leave the money exchange out of your Pilates sessions. This will make your client feel even better and more relaxed.

Special Rates

In the beginning of this chapter, I told you that raising prices is one of the hardest things for any business to do. For exactly this reason, I strongly recommend not to give special rates at all.

That's easy to say, but let's face it: There are situations where you'll feel that it is the right thing to do. No successful studio I know of can avoid having a few exceptions to the official pricing policy. There might be an injured dancer who wants to work with you but is already living on a tight budget. If you have ever worked as a dancer, you know this situation all too well and will be tempted to help this person in pain. There might be someone who is the sweetest person you know but does not have enough to pay your private rate, and you simply can't turn this person down. There might be a long-time client who suddenly becomes unemployed but wants to continue his or her training.

In each of these cases, you have to ask yourself how you feel about the individual case and whether you can afford to give a special rate. Again, raising the price later on will be hard, so whenever you end up giving a special rate to someone, you have to be very clear that:

- The special rate is only temporary, you can call it off at any time

- Payments must be made on the day of each class or ahead of time

Remember that giving a class at a special rate will cost you income. Try to limit your special prices to two clients at most.

Pricing checklist:

✔ Don't offer "introductory rates."

✔ Any first class is free of charge. After that, you and the client decide if you want to work with each other.

✔ Don't do walk-ins for mat classes... period.

✔ Don't do the scheduling for semi-privates. This is up to your clients.

✔ Get cash out of the way—offer discounted class cards.

✔ Limit the number of special-rate clients to two.

Accounting

Here is a quick overview on accounting: Your core skill is being an excellent Pilates teacher with a lot of knowledge in the field of mind-body exercise—you don't have to be an accountant. Don't burden yourself with a complicated computer accounting system or daily bookkeeping. It will be a pain, and you might lose interest and stop finding your business fun altogether.

Most Pilates trainers I have known do their own basic accounting by keeping index cards for each client. They will pencil in when the client takes a class, what issues and health conditions the client has, and when a class card was paid for. One index card will most likely carry you through a full year with this client. At the end of the year, you can simply put all the information into an Excel spreadsheet and do a cross-check with your bank account. Your golden rule for accounting should be "KISS"—keep it short and simple!

When transferring data from the index cards to your Excel spreadsheet, you should focus on the dates when your clients have seen you and when you received payment from them. In the beginning, it will give you some extra security if you do your client accounting at the end of every month.

You should also put all your expenses into an Excel spreadsheet on a monthly basis. By doing this, you keep perfect control of your costs. Keep your receipts for each month in a separate envelope, and enter them into the sheet at the end of each month.

If you do your accounting correctly, the balance between all your expenses and all the client payments should match your bank account. Be sure to get yourself at least a basic business checking account to keep all your Pilates space finances separate from your private finances. Be careful with the class cards that you might offer. You will receive payment long before you actually give the class, so don't get confused by this fact when trying to balance your bank account against your income statement.

Whether or not you hire a CPA, you may have to get used to taking care of some basic accounting. As long as you keep careful records and make a good effort to stay organized, you will be surprised how simple this task can be!

Just in case this chapter has left you asking whether anybody will really spend money on privates, the answer is: **Yes, they will!**

You will have regular group classes for those who cannot afford privates (or do not want to spend the money), and then there are the wealthy people in every community who will expect a special environment and treatment for their money. The fact that you have a small boutique studio can be your greatest asset. Then, there are always people who choose to make the investment (even if they are not wealthy) because attending to their bodies truly means something to them.

How easy is it to spend $30,000 on a car and not even think about it? The $50 to $95 your clients will pay per session will probably not stay in their pockets if they cut out Pilates. In fact, it will probably go toward something that is not nearly as beneficial to them or important to their health and happiness.

Remember, you are not selling tight abs or buff arms. You are on a mission to help people find a connection with dynamic alignment and a healthy lifestyle. It is the connection they pay for, which is ultimately an investment back into themselves. We are just facilitators of a much greater journey.

Schedule	Monday	Tuesday	Wednesday	Thursday	Friday	Saturday	Sunday
7AM	Reserved for private client/summer class	Reserved for private client/summer class	Reserved for private client/summer class	Reserved for private client/summer class	Reserved for private client/summer class	Reserved for private client/summer class	Rental
8AM	Intermediate Mat and Small Apparatus	Private	Intermediate Mat and Small Apparatus	Private	Advanced Mat	Open Mat	Rental
9AM	Private	Private	Private	Private	Private	Open Mat	Rental
10AM	Private	Beginning Mat	Private	Intermediate Mat and Small Apparatus	Private	Pilates on Ball	Rental
11AM	Private	Private	Private	Private	Advanced Mat	Private	Rental
12PM	Intermediate Mat and Small Apparatus		Intermediate Mat and Small Apparatus			Power Pilates	Rental
1PM			Off/Rental				Rental
2PM			Off/Rental				Rental
3PM	Private		Off/Rental		Private		Rental
4PM	Private	Private	Off/Rental	Private	Duet		Rental
5PM	Private		Off/Rental				Rental
6PM	Pilates on the Ball	Power Pilates Mat	Off/Rental	Power Pilates Mat			Rental
7PM			Off/Rental				
8PM							
9PM							
10PM							

DEVELOPING A PRICING STRATEGY

Notes:

Making the Most of Your Time

Scheduling is crucial, yet I'd bet that nobody even brought it up during your training. Am I correct?

The type of Pilates studio that we are advocating here—extra small, with a predetermined number of available client sessions—calls for strategic scheduling. What is a good strategy?

You have to set your priorities carefully. As you will see, a good strategy for a small Pilates studio differs significantly from a good strategy for a large fitness center that sells memberships and is open late every night in order to accommodate the needs of its clients.

Before we start discussing priorities in detail, I want to share two pieces of advice that I doubt anyone who is in the business of selling Pilates certifications or equipment will tell you. Those people in particular are likely to tell you some long-standing myths in the industry: You need lots of space, and group classes will generate revenue. Here's some alternative advice:

- You must give your private clients priority. Once a time on a particular day is built into their schedules, they are very likely to stick with it for years. They not only provide your steady income, but they are more loyal to you than a person in a large group class will ever be. The intensity of a private lesson and the intimacy, trust, and even friendship that comes with it makes that time of the day a safe haven for both you and your client. It is much more personal, important, and worth protecting than you may think.

- Group classes do not necessarily make money. They never make money for the small studio. You need to have a very large studio indeed (think 20 Reformers in one of several rooms) to create the kind of hype that could make such a class profitable. And even if that is the case, imagine how much cash you have to come up with to buy all that equipment. Imagine how much advertising you would have to do to get the word out. Unless you treat mat classes like semi-privates (five people max) and sell class packages for eight or ten weeks that will make clients commit to the group, you are losing money. Again, in semi-private classes, the social aspect comes into play: the group grows close and progresses together, which make people feel more loyal to the class and to you. If five people pay $15 per class ahead of time, you walk out with $75 per hour even if not everyone shows up. Not bad, is it?

These guidelines give you a couple more reasons why a large space can actually work against you. People may rent a bigger, more expensive space thinking that it will attract ten people who will commit to a mat class. This is not going to happen. It is more likely that the studio will gather a lax group of students who show up whenever they feel like it. And on top of all that, it is difficult to focus on bringing in and keeping private clients.

Remember: **Fewer people means a higher level of individual commitment**. They know that if they don't show up, everybody in the group will notice. "Where is Diane? Let's call her; let's hassle her. Why did she miss class?" Bingo.

Now that we have cleared that up, let's look at how you are going to organize your available working hours into a strategic schedule. Why not start creating the perfect schedule right now? Use the worksheet at the end of this chapter to make the most out of the following list.

Priority 1: YOU

Sit down and think about when you feel your best. Are you an early bird or a night owl? Do you have kids to take to or pick up from school on certain days of the week? Do you have any personal commitments that you don't want to give up?

Block out those times and days on the Your Schedule worksheet at the end of this chapter. Now you are left with times and days that agree with your energy level and fit in with other commitments.

Priority 2: Give the Client Options

Now, spread out your available working hours into different parts of the week. I would suggest that if you plan to work part time, you schedule three back-to-back hours in the late morning and a mat class late afternoon, Monday through Thursday. Take Friday off and consider adding some extra hours on Saturday morning.

Make sure that you have either:

1. Three long mornings teaching a block of four hours and two short afternoons teaching two hours;

2. Three short afternoons and two long mornings; or

3. Four long mornings (including Saturday) and two short afternoons.

If that does not work with your other commitments, then choose a different schedule. There are potential clients who have availability in their schedules at any time of the day or night—you just need to find them. The point is: Match clients to your schedule, not vice versa.

Priority 3: Privates & Mat Classes

Invest most, if not all, your energy into recruiting private clients. They should constitute the bulk of your income. Then add mat classes to open up the studio to people who are not sure that they want to invest in private sessions or cannot afford them. Here is a general rule of thumb in terms of distribution:

Half-Time Teaching (18 hours/week)	Full-Time Teaching (25 hours/week)	Full-Time+ Teaching (30 hours/week)
14 Privates	19 Privates	23 Privates
1 Semi-private	2 Semi-privates	2 Semi-privates
3 Mat classes	4 Mat classes	5 Mat classes

When you schedule mat classes, keep in mind that people should have the chance to work out twice per week if they would like to. It makes sense to offer beginning mat classes, for example, on two non-consecutive days at the same time. Ten weeks later, you could offer intermediate mat classes at the same times and build in a new beginning class on the other days. Once you have started to build up your clientele, do not change what works unless you absolutely have to. They will become used to your class schedule and organize their lives to accommodate it. People seek that stability.

As a general rule, I would suggest that group classes work best in the early evening (starting from 5:00 to 7:00 PM) or at lunchtime (12:30 PM). If you have a very limited amount of space, you can also try a 10:00 or 11:00 AM mat class if you find three or four people who are willing to commit to it ahead of time.

Tip: In the beginning, we are tempted to try to accommodate every client who comes our way. Avoid it if possible. If you are too obliging, you are basically training your new clients that they can come and work out any time of day or night and on weekends, and they will expect this in the future. Stick to your own schedule; it will work out better in the end.

Priority 4: Renting Space to Others

Renting out space should not be a means to make a profit; it just reduces your overhead and keeps your studio busy. Make sure to leave good times available for renting the space when you create your schedule. There is no point in offering space for rent if you are blocking all the prime time. Give renters an excellent deal so they stick with you. You may choose to rent out space to other Pilates teachers or to different types of mind-body practitioners. If you have a small room, it could be good for massage. You may decide to rent out your main space to Feldenkrais practiconers, Alexander teachers, or yoga instructors.

I often see that experienced Pilates teachers want to rent out their space to other Pilates teachers for an arm and a leg. Here is the deal: You either rent space to someone who is very good for relatively little money, or you rent space to someone who is young and inexperienced for a lot of money. Why? The experienced teacher has no need to give you half of her income. That teacher could do it herself, around the corner, and all of a sudden you have a competitor. Or, that teacher gets a great deal from you, does not have to invest in equipment, and makes your studio the best in town. Think about it. Which would you rather have? I like renting out space for a nominal fee to my teacher friends. It is important that you trust the person renting from you.

On the other hand, the inexperienced instructor will gladly accept the high rent for the chance to practice in a professional atmosphere. But, if that instructor is good, he or she may very well decide to do his or her own thing around the corner from your studio next year. (Do you see the pattern here?) If you make the mistake of hiring a bad teacher who is willing to pay you high rent, you are asking for a headache. That teacher's clients will not stay, the teacher will moan and groan constantly, and you have to deal with a bad reputation.

On a more positive note, working alongside someone you like is a lot of fun as well. At the Movement Center, my partner Aimee McDonald and I sometimes crack up laughing about our teaching habits or when we crash into each other hunting for equipment that one of us has hidden in a different place. On a good week, the two of us see 60 clients in four tiny rooms.

A good schedule of standing appointments will become ingrained in your life. I can't imagine a Wednesday morning at 8:00 without my client Jenny or a Thursday evening without Pat. People seek stability. This holds true for clients just as much as it does for teachers!

WORKSHEET: YOUR SCHEDULE

Schedule	Monday	Tuesday	Wednesday
7:00AM			
8:00AM			
9:00AM			
10:00AM			
11:00AM			
12:00PM			
1:00PM			
2:00PM			
3:00PM			
4:00PM			
5:00PM			
6:00PM			
7:00PM			
8:00PM			
9:00PM			
10:00PM			

Thursday	Friday	Saturday	Sunday

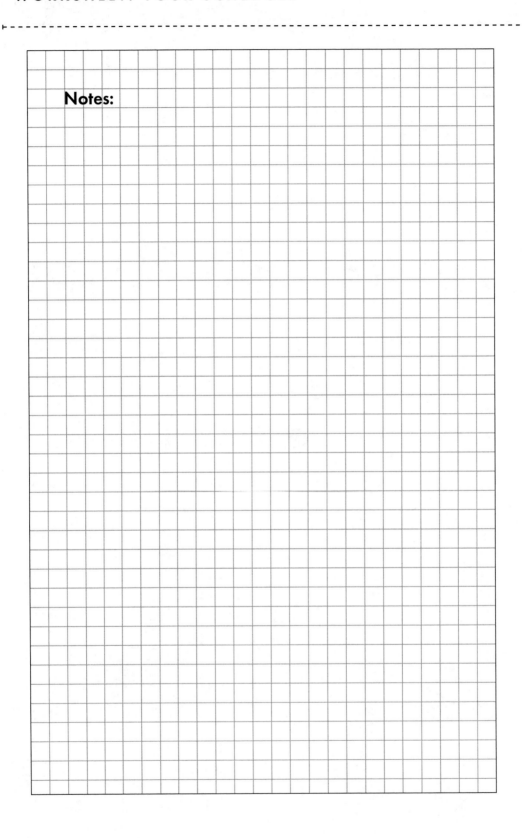

Notes:

Creativity and Vision

CHAPTER TEN

HOLLY FURGASON

You worked day and night for a year—possibly even longer—to open your studio. You found the perfect location, negotiated the lease, purchased beautiful equipment, freshly painted the walls, and stocked the bathroom with fancy soap and lotion. You turn over the "Open" sign and expect to see a flood of clients rush into your space. But after a few weeks, there is still no one banging down your door. Your initial excitement turns to concern.

You know you need to promote your business, but where do you begin? How do you get the word out?

This chapter lays out a strategy that will help you get started at promoting you studio effectively. You will need to set aside time for self-promotion so that you can establish a sales strategy, decide how best to implement your strategy, and design your studio's identity.

Designating Time for Marketing

Promotion is critical for any successful studio, and creating effective promotional material will take a significant amount of time. Experts suggest that you should develop a weekly time commitment to marketing. Depending on the number of clients you hope (or need) to generate, you should spend 5% to 40% of your work week promoting your business. Because this is a huge amount of time that you will be investing in marketing, you do not want to be haphazard in your efforts.

Decide what is reasonable for your schedule. Write these hours into your planner so that you are truly committed to spending structured time on marketing each and every week until your studio is well established.

Establishing a Sales Strategy

Developing a simple sales strategy will help you focus your marketing efforts and capital more effectively during the start-up stage of your studio. A sales strategy is basically a list of sales goals and objectives. The specific details of your sales strategy should reflect your Pilates philosophy and articulate the goals that are important to you.

Start by asking yourself questions that help you clarify the needs of your market, determine the type of clientele you are seeking, and identify the competitive differences that create a place for you in your local market.

- Do you seek mainly private, semi-private, or group class clients?

- What is the average age of the clients you seek?

- What do the studios in your area offer?

- What do the studios in your area lack?

- Can you serve a special population that is currently not being served? For example, will you focus on rehabilitation, pregnancy, or serious athletes?

- What can you offer that provides the client with a unique experience? Do you offer conveniences such as free parking, showers, or open mat classes, or service-oriented extras such as workshops, teacher trainings, experienced staff, or on-site massage?

Write a few sentences that clearly state these key features. As your business grows, revisit these statements and assess how you are meeting the objectives you outlined.

Implementing Your Sales Strategy

You have three main opportunities through which you can implement your sales strategy: networking, referrals, and advertising. Creating balance among these approaches is key.

Networking

You should research and explore other businesses in your area that could complement the services you offer. For example, it is great to cultivate relationships with businesses that offer chiropractic treatment, massage therapy, acupuncture, physical therapy, and running and triathlon training. Introduce yourself to these business owners, and if your philosophies align, discuss a referral agreement that could benefit both your businesses and your clients' needs. Instituting casual partnerships with industry leaders in your area creates a web of businesses that refer clients to you. Aligning your studio with the best of the local body workers helps you create a professional image.

Referrals

The most cost-effective way to advertise your business is through client referrals. Nothing speaks more favorably for your business then a happy client telling others about his or her wonderful experience at your studio. And the best part is that it does not cost you a dime!

Consider devising a rewards scheme to thank clients for referring their friends to your studio, such as a free foam roller or a percentage off the purchase of a private package.

Advertising

Many new studios spend all their initial time and energy on print advertising—everything from promotional postcards to advertisements in local newspapers. There is no question that print advertising will help inform the public that your studio exists, but the rate of return is often difficult to determine. Also keep in mind that in order to find out any advertising statistics, you must ask all your new clients how they heard about your studio and keep record of this information. Because of these factors, print advertising should not be your primary means of promoting your new business. However, some well planned advertisements may bring in new clients.

Instead of going for larger publications, look in your community for smaller advertising options such as neighborhood newspapers or specialty papers. This may allow you to speak more directly to your target population, and it may also get you a larger piece of the publication's real estate for less money.

According to Cameron Foote in *The Business Side of Creativity*, studies show that advertising tends to pay off if the ad is run multiple times. The more times you run the ad, the more likely you will pay for the cost of the ad. When determining the cost of running an advertisement, you should think of it as a year-long commitment even if you have the option to renew each month. "As a rule of thumb, kill any ad or campaign with a rate of return on investment of less than 2 to 1; increase the frequency of any ad or campaign with a ratio of more than 2 to 1," suggests Foote.

Because of the high cost of producing and running an ad, you want to be sure that it has significant content. What is significant with regard to your studio will depend on your philosophy and your sales goals. Regardless of the specifics of these goals, good writing is critical for marketing material. As movement people, we do not spend a lot of time writing, and many studio owners experience writer's block when it comes to putting their thoughts about their studios down on paper. But it is important to think carefully about what your advertisements will say to the public. Simply putting an ad out there isn't enough.

Recently, a business owner asked me to develop an ad for a local newspaper. When I asked for the text that would be in the ad, the studio owner said that she just thought she would pull something off her Web site. It is not worth spending $2000 or even $200 dollars to run an ad when the text has not been well conceived. Imagine you could have a phone conversation with every potential dream client. What would you say? Print advertising gives you the chance to do just that—state your mission, what is unique about you, and what you love. Be creative and use your imagination.

Designing Your Identity

After you have developed a sales strategy, you should have a better understanding of your studio's identity, and therefore a better understanding of how you should represent yourself visually.

You know your business better than anyone else does, and therefore your active participation is fundamental to the design process. Creating a studio identity will define your relationship with potential clients and give them key information about the types of services you can provide for them.

Working with a designer is highly collaborative, and therefore, you should employ a designer who is interested in this line of work, who has an appreciation for movement, and with whom you feel comfortable. The graphic designer you retain should be seen as a creative resource; you don't have to know exactly what you want because he or she will guide you through the design process.

In the beginning, most new studio owners cannot afford to produce all their marketing materials. However, you want to lay down a strong foundation for your studio's visual identity. Your studio's marketing schedule can be divided into two design phases. The first phase should be implemented when you open your studio, and the second step by step over time.

Design Phase One:

On a small budget of $800, this first design phase can produce the essential elements necessary for the success of your new studio: a logo, signage, business cards, and a flyer/brochure/schedule.

Logo

A logo should reaffirm your philosophy visually. You may have a very clear picture in your head for your business's logo, from the color and placement of the text to the details of the illustration. Or you may not have a clue how to represent your business graphically. Both approaches are perfectly acceptable to any good graphic designer.

Depending on the amount of money you spend, the designer will produce one or more logo prototypes for you. Collectively, you and your designer will hone in the design that best communicates your business philosophy. Make sure it is something you can live with—it should follow your sense of style and business décor, and you should be able to see it printed on studio signage or merchandise such as T-shirts and water bottles.

What makes a good logo?

- It is immediately recognizable.

- It conveys the studio philosophy, ethos, and mission.

- It will look good very small (1/2 inch) or very large (15 feet).

- It is timeless, not trendy. (Will it look dated in five years?)

Tip: Collect ideas or examples of things you like. A page torn from a magazine, scribblings on a cocktail napkin, or a business card from a competitor can be creative inspiration to you and your designer. Place them in a folder, and take them to your design consultation.

Signage

You are not in business unless you have a sign. There are many options in business signage that range drastically in price—window stickers, menu boards, banners. Be sure to check with city regulations and your landlord before having a sign built or printed. I once made a sign for a studio that ended up in a closet because it did not meet city regulations.

- Make sure it can be read from a distance.

- Ask the printer how the color will match your existing color scheme. If you think it will print orange and it ends up pink, there could be some problems.

- Keep the text to a minimum—business name and possibly a street or Web address.

- Your sign will help reinforce your studio's identity.

- The sign should blend nicely with the building's architecture.

Business cards

Business cards may be your first contact with potential clients. Because of this, you should put some extra effort into producing top-notch, professional cards.

How can I make nice business cards without spending a fortune?

- Finding a good printer is essential. One way to do this is to collect business cards that you like and find out who printed them.

- Stick with the standard size card (2 x 3.5 inches) and standard weight card stock, and use minimal color. Thicker, colored, or textured paper, printing on both sides, and printing multiple colors will cost a premium. Decide what is essential to the image you wish to present and what is just icing on the cake. If you are developing a newer studio, ask yourself what you can live without until the studio is fully established.

- If possible, print your cards in bulk. Most printers have price breaks when printing 500 or more cards at a time.

TIP: Once your business cards are printed, carry them with you in a cardholder, planner, or wallet pocket. Digging around in your bag to pull out a worn card with bent corners is a poor representation of your business and a waste of the money spent to produce clean, crisp cards.

Flyer/Brochure/Schedule

In the start-up stage of your studio, you should combine these three marketing pieces into one. This single printed piece can be distributed inexpensively, contains information about studio philosophy, services offered, and rates, and provides a schedule of group classes.

It is a good idea to create a template for this all-inclusive piece. With very little time, you can insert new material into your template easily for distribution—from special class offerings and studio announcements to rate changes and new services. The easiest way to produce a professional yet flexible template is to have a designer produce a layout in a program you own, such as Microsoft Word or Microsoft Publisher, so that you can use it over and over again. You can also opt to use one of the templates that normally comes in these software programs.

I can't tell you how many times I have heard a studio owner say, "We have a change in our class schedule (or staff or rates or services or Web address), but I just had 1000 brochures printed!" A template is the best way to avoid this scenario. The template allows you to make the changes yourself instead of going through the graphic designer.

You can also print fewer pieces more frequently so that the information is current. Once you are well established, you can work on something more permanent.

What makes a good basic flyer/brochure/schedule?

- Your logo and business name are clearly presented.

- The colors used will look good posted around your studio.

- It looks clean printed in black and white or in full color.

- It doesn't need to be cut or trimmed.

- Be consistent with your identity.

- The schedule is easy to navigate and understandable at a glance.

- Find a location in your studio and always have it stocked with the current schedule. Clients will get used to picking it up there.

TIP: Negative space is important. Try to create a balance between empty space and filled space on your flyer/brochure/schedule. You want to give the text, images, and graphics room to breathe, but you don't want the page to look empty.

Design Phase Two:

The Web site, letterhead, photography, posters, postcards, and swag are really not essential in the beginning. It is tempting to want to produce these things early on because they are fun, but really think about the bottom line.

Web site

You may be surprised to see a Web site in the second design phase. There are several reasons for this. In order to see the information on the site, the prospective client must know the address or specifically seek out the information provided. This means that you have to advertise your Web site (which is essentially what you are doing when you list it on business cards, flyers, etc.). Another problem with thinking of a Web site as a primary marketing tool is that a Web site cannot target people who would be particularly receptive to your services.

Just like it takes time to establish a reputation as an instructor, it takes time to establish a presence on the Web. As your business gets more well known in your community, and as you establish your network with other business owners, other people will link to you. This will help generate traffic to your site. You can think of getting Internet traffic like panning for gold—other businesses that are aligned with Pilates will filter out the people who wouldn't be interested in bodywork, leaving only the potential customers. Your Web site will shift from being a soft marketing tool to a strong promotional resource, but this will take time. It is impossible to buy this reputation.

Many new Web site owners are tempted by the advertisements that promise more traffic. However, this may not be the traffic you want. Keep in mind that simply because you are on the Web doesn't mean that you will generate new clients. You have the choice: either build a reputation over time, or speed up the process with a greater financial investment. If you pay for more traffic, you may end up with fool's gold.

If you feel that you absolutely have to have a Web site right from the start, a good compromise would be to use an inexpensive computer program to build a single page. Usually, one of these programs will come with your operating system. This simple page should act as a sort of online version of your flyer/brochure/schedule.

Remember that good design involves much more than simply being able to put information on the Web, so when you are ready to build a full Web site, I recommend retaining a designer. The professional site you will end up with will be worth it.

What makes a good Web site?

- Provide information or usable content—not just a beautiful site.
- A Web site is useless if the information contained on it is outdated. Update your content frequently.
- Navigation and the overall usability of the site is the key to helping viewers find information.
- Optimize graphics, images, and special content for the Web.
- Start with a basic site, and then add functionality over time.

When you are ready to build a full Web site, you should do some planning to organize your thoughts before meeting with your designer.

First, you must define the goals and objectives for the site. Some examples of objectives include recruiting new clients, creating a sense of studio community, and providing information or additional resources on techniques offered. Take the time to think about your Web site goals, and then clearly and concisely articulate them on paper.

Second, you must define your audience. Is this site for current clients, prospective clients, trainers, trainees, or some other audience group? Probably, it will be a mixture of all these groups, but depending on your goals, it may need to be weighted more heavily toward one group or another. Write down your audience groups and then rank them according to importance.

Third, make a list of reasons why you think each audience group would be coming to your site. For example, a new mom might come to the site to check class schedules, rates, and information about postpartum training. Your Web site should aim to address all of the needs of each of your audience groups.

Your Web site goals, the ranked list of audiences, and the list of reasons why various visitors would come to your site will be invaluable resources during all stages of the design build. They will help you and the designer stay on track, and they will ensure that you won't be disappointed with the end product.

Tip: Go online and find examples of mind-body Web sites that you like in terms of overall look. Make a list of these sites and include simple comments stating what you like about each site. Don't forget to ask permission to use any graphics or photos you find on the Internet, in books, or in magazines.

Letterhead

Before you run out and print several reams of letterhead, consider how it will be used. Many studios do much of their correspondence with clients via email, on the telephone, or in person. Ask yourself if it worth the cost of printing and if an electronic version of letterhead would suffice.

How can I make an electronic studio letterhead?

- Have your logo designer give you a version of your logo that is large (in size and resolution).

- Insert the logo into the header or footer of a document. Type in other useful text such as contact information and save it as a template.

Photography

Few things scream "amateur" louder than bad photography. Good photography takes time and practice. Start shooting everything! Over time, you will have a significant number of quality photos at your disposal.

Before shooting, be sure to ask permission from your subjects, preferably in writing, to keep on file. It is not a good idea to just take photos of a group class and post them on the studio's Web site. It is bad etiquette and could lead to a lawsuit. Think of how you feel when a photographer shows up unexpectedly: Is my outfit okay? Is my hair a mess? What are these pictures for and who is going to see them? How embarrassing! Typically, clients are willing, and even flattered, to be included, if they are asked first.

What will make my photos look more professional?

- If using a digital camera, capture the images at the highest resolution available.

- Scan the photos at a minimum of 300 dpi (dots per inch). This gives the designer more flexibility.

- Lighting is arguably more important than the camera itself. It doesn't make sense to use photos of poorly lit figures doing indeterminate exercises on your marketing material.

- Simplify backgrounds by removing unnecessary objects that distract from the subject.

- Use a tripod.

Tip: Find examples of photographs that you like in magazines or online, identify what it is you like about the images, and then without copying the original photograph, try to recreate aspects such as setting and lighting in your own studio.

Posters and postcards

Glossy, full color postcards, and sturdy, large-format posters can be very effective marketing tools. However, they also can be costly. You want to design a piece that you can print in large quantities and distribute over time for special purposes.

How do I future-proof my posters and postcards?

- The information should not be liable to change. Really think about the essential content so you don't end up throwing them away after six months because the information is no longer applicable.

- Make sure your studio's name and contact information is prominent.

Tip: Think about posters and postcards as ways to advertise your studio in general more than a single event or technique at cafes, restaurants, laundromats, and businesses.

Pilates Philosophy:

_____
_____
_____
_____

Mission:

_____
_____
_____
_____

☑ Sales Strategy:

_____
_____
_____
_____
_____
_____

☐ Networking opportunities:

_____
_____
_____
_____

☐ Referrals

☐ Advertising opportunities:

_____
_____
_____
_____

Studio Identity ☑

Logo ☐

Signage ☐

Business cards ☐

Flyer/Brochure/Schedule ☐

☑ **Final Tips:**

☐ Graphic designers are expensive, but the beauty of Pilates is that you can trade almost any service for classes. If trading is out of the question, graphic designers' hourly fees are typically representative of their training, experience, and creativity, and, in most cases, the amount of effort they are willing to put into you and your project.

☐ Designers are not proofreaders. Make sure YOU see a proof of all printed material. It would be a disaster to print 500 business cards with the wrong address.

☐ Strive to be clear, clean, and simple. Design does not need to be complex to be effective and make an impact. Good design should inform and facilitate communication.

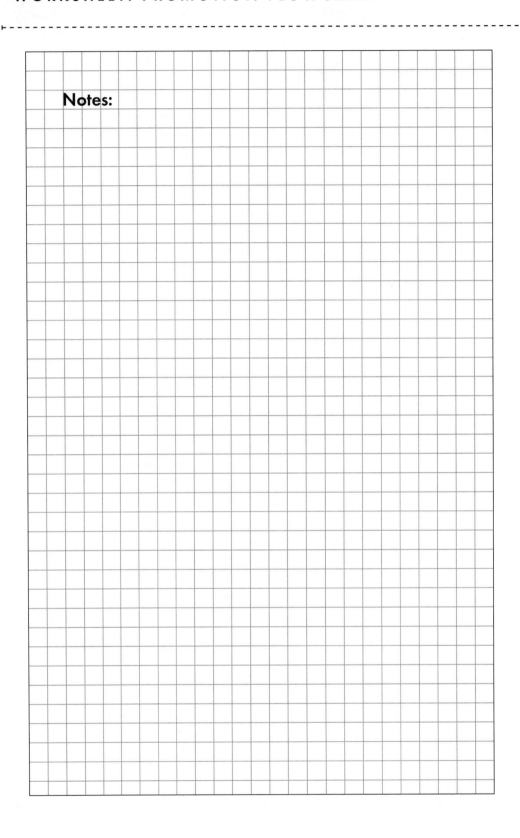

Notes:

Five Ways to Keep Your Clients Coming Back

CHAPTER ELEVEN

Matchmaking

Think eBay and the success of matchmaking on a global level. You may be the perfect person to teach a certain individual. This relationship will be fruitful, satisfying, long lasting, and motivating. It will keep you taking the type of work approach you love and do best. Since word of mouth is the best referral, you are very likely to keep meeting people who are similar to your existing clients. A community is born!

Send a press kit to your local newspaper, radio, and TV station (see Chapter 10 on marketing). Have an open house with free classes. Teach for free at any event you can get into before the grand opening of your studio, whether it is a church, a community center, a dance studio, or a school. Send flyers to all health professionals in your immediate area and offer a free session to them so they can get to know your work. These health professionals include massage therapists, chiropractors, orthopedic surgeons, and most importantly, physical therapists. A good network of referrals is essential, and everybody will benefit from it.

One way of initiating an excellent client relationship is to assess motivation and keep revisiting it in your new therapeutic relationship.

Usually it all starts with a phone call.

First Phone Call

Nancy Hodari, owner of the STOTT PILATES™ certification center Equilibrium in Bloomfield Hills, Michigan, feels that the first contact with a studio or teacher is so important that she invested in a receptionist right away. "People want to speak with a human being about something as personal as their bodies and workout plans," she says.

Playing phone tag for days is the reality of my own teaching life in a small studio. My phone is off when I teach, which is several hours per day, and then the phone tag begins. This may not seem very professional or "consumer friendly," but I don't have much of a choice, and clients understand that I will be calling them back as soon as I can. I find that email works well for scheduling and answering clients' questions. I try to get to it twice a day. Of course, if a client needs to cancel at the last minute, there is no alternative but to call my cell phone. Most of the time, these calls are urgent. I find that potential new clients usually prefer to email anyway, so this system works for me and for my clients.

You must be prepared. You have to know what you are going to ask the new client, how you will present your approach to fitness, and how you will discuss finances, all of which you should discuss in your first conversation. That way, your first session can be spent focusing on the client, because you will have already addressed your approach and studio policy.

I always feel uncomfortable when I go to a studio and the first thing they tell me is: "The class is 15 bucks and you need to fill out all these forms." Don't run one of those studios!

Take notes while you are on the phone or right afterward; it is very helpful to remember information such as whether the client has injuries and why he or she is interested in Pilates, as well as personal information such as whether the client has kids or the client's hobbies for initiating your first meeting.

Free Sessions?

There are a lot of takes on whether a free initial session is a useful marketing tool to get people in the door. I believe it is, as I've mentioned before. However, I do not like the label "trial class," since it makes me feel like someone is about to be sentenced. I offer a free "coaching class" in which the client and I both assess whether we can work together. The class involves some talking about background information, some postural analysis that I share with the client by way of digital photographs, and then a good workout.

After certifying, I was so hung up on the principles of Pilates that clients would have to sit through an hour of in-depth discussion about the pelvis. They would leave frustrated and never come back. Clients are there to move, not to hear us talk! They can get a video for that.

Motivation

Motivation is pretty much a given when a client enters the studio. That person has jumped through several hoops already—he or she has asked around for a good Pilates teacher, made an appointment, and taken time out of his or her busy schedule. The person coming through your door is not a blank slate; he or she is motivated to try something new.

It is important to discern two types of motivation: extrinsic and intrinsic. Extrinsically motivated people need outside rewards to keep their motivation alive. They are the clients who will specifically address things they would like you to help them accomplish: fix this or that, tone up or down, lose weight, relieve pain, and so forth.

Intrinsically motivated individuals do not need outside rewards to keep doing what they like or what feels good. They find the strength of persistence within themselves—they are the ones who will do the exercises at home and come back to the studio every time with a new discovery. These are also high achievers who want to get better and will work for it.

Keeping clients motivated is a balancing act. You will need to compromise and program in such a way that they feel listened to, while slowly educating them about the others issues you would like to see addressed at the same time. Here are five ways to keep them coming back to you:

1. Client Assessment: Priorities

Do you want to get out of pain?

Do you want to change your physical appearance? (Do you want to lose weight or improve posture?)

Do you want to take time for yourself to unwind?

Do you want to try Pilates because it is popular?

2. Self-Assessment: Do the client's priorities match yours?

Do I see completely different priorities from the client?

Is the client unaware of certain aspects of Pilates training that I deem to be important?

If you answer "yes" to either of these self-assessment questions, you will have to hold back on your needs and address the client's priorities first so he or she feels listened to. Then start the educational process and bring up your suggestions one at a time. The client will see this as a challenge for growth and take it on with pleasure.

3. Build Your Argument

When meeting a client for the first time, it is important to choose a time of the day when you are not tired or worn out. Seeing new clients at the beginning of the week is good way to encourage them to make another appointment that same week, giving them the chance to get into a routine and giving you the opportunity to build up the relationship.

Training once a week, especially in the beginning, will make it difficult to deliver what the method promises. It is important that we are clear about this with our clients. You will have to answer the ever-popular question: How long does it take before I see results? The question itself calls for some explanation. Usually I say: "We are trying to balance out a 40-hour work week, where you may be sitting on your tailbone all day long, with 60 minutes of training once per week. The odds are stacked 40 to 1 against us. Give us some time, ideally one private and one mat class per week. You will notice results in how you look and feel pretty rapidly. Even doing the exercises 15 minutes a day in your home does wonders for your body's muscle memory and readiness."

4. Pacing: Getting it just right

After we have enquired about the client's broad priorities, it is our job as trainers to narrow down these priorities to manageable chunks without sacrificing the intellectual stimulation necessary to keep our clients interested.

In psychology, this process is called pacing. Pacing essentially makes up the qualitative element in your programming. If the pacer is too low, exercises are constantly repeated without variations (which is a common problem with big mat classes or if you teach strictly by the book), motivation declines, and clients get bored. If the pacer is too high, however, you are dealing out new exercises and more difficult variations than the client can handle. Clients may get frustrated and not come back.

5. Feedback

We should ask for clients' feedback regularly. The easiest way is to provide anonymous forms and install a drop box. You can ask questions about the appearance of the studio, clients' future goals with mind-body fitness, and if they would like to be videotaped once in a while. There is nothing like visual feedback for people to make instant corrections. We should not forget that most clients will never have seen themselves doing Pilates exercises. So their perception may be very different from their actual execution of the exercise.

Also, conduct mini planning sessions for future goals. A client of mine once told me: "I have been in a Pilates mat class for three years now. On the walls, I see the charts that say 'Essential,' 'Intermediate,' and 'Advanced.' Nobody ever talked to me about where I am, what needs to improve, and how I get to the advanced level."

This is a totally understandable concern. We are competitive animals, and if I hang up a poster that divides exercises into levels, it is normal for my clients to aspire to that. Announce your clients' progress. Often it is hard for them to tell whether they are progressing when you keep doing similar things, and assessing progress is important in keeping people motivated.

Clients' feedback is their wish list. Feedback motivates us to address their new needs;

we have a responsibility to do so. If we identify our clients' priorities and gear our teaching toward them, we will see progress and witness a motivational boost unlike anything we've ever imagined.

Timeline:
Putting It All Together

TIMELINE: PUTTING IT ALL TOGETHER

12-6 Months Before

- [ ] Determine whether this is the right time to open your own studio
- [ ] Decide if you want to work with a partner or on your own
- [ ] Visit other studios and take notes
- [ ] Start collecting design samples
- [ ] Meet with a lawyer
- [ ] Choose your partner and start talking about your partnership agreement

6-4 Months Before

- [ ] Tell your current employer you are moving on
- [ ] Write a mission statement
- [ ] Find the right area for your studio
- [ ] Scout out the perfect Pilates space
- [ ] Research pricing for Pilates equipment and manufacturers
- [ ] Find potential advertising venues or publications and request pricing info
- [ ] Draft a partnership agreement
- [ ] Hire a CPA

2 Months Before

- [ ] Start calling equipment manfacturers to negotiate discounts
- [ ] Hire a graphic designer
- [ ] Make sure your studio name is clear for use
- [ ] Finalize your studio name
- [ ] Register a domain name with your studio name
- [ ] Begin designing a logo, sinage, and business cards
- [ ] Develop an advertising strategy
- [ ] Design advertisements
- [ ] Start to think about when you want to schedule classes

1 Month Before

☐ Negotiate your lease

☐ Renovate and decorate your space

☐ Purchase large equipment and small apparatus

☐ Get insurance

☐ Finalize your class schedule

☐ Begin designing a flyer/brochure/schedule

☐ Prepare client intake forms and liability waiver

☐ Check with your local newspaper and see if it will run a story about your new business

2 - 1 Weeks Before

☐ Purchase appliances and supplies

☐ Call utility companies to set up phone line, water, electricity, and Internet

After Your Studio Is Up and Running

☐ Hire a cleaning service

☐ Actively seek out network of mind-body professionals

☐ Plan for a grand opening celebration

☐ Arrange for other mind-body professionals to rent out your space

☐ Begin photographing studio events, classes, etc.

☐ Begin designing Web site, letterhead, and posters

☐ Celebrate your milestones

☐ Build on your Pilates equipment

Notes:

References

Conraths-Lange, Nicola. *Survival Skills for Pilates Teachers*. Ann Arbor: Logokinesis Publishing, 2004.

Deering, Anne and Anne Murphy. *The Partnering Imperative: Making Business Partnerships Work*. Hoboken: John Whiley & Sons Publishers, 2003.

Edwards, Sarah and Paul Edwards. *Working from Home: Everything you need to know about living and working under the same roof*. New York: Penguin Putnam Inc., 2004.

FindLaw for Business. "Creating a Partnership Agreement." http://biz.findlaw.com/business.

Foote, Cameron. *The Business Side of Creativity*. New York: W. W. Norton & Company, Inc., 2002.

Gardner, Howard. *Frames of Mind: The Theory of Multiple Intelligences*. New York: Basic Books, 1983.

Gonzalez, Maria. "A Practical Guide to Alliances," *Ivey Business Journal*. Ontario: Ivey Publishing, Vol 66:Issue 1, 2001.

Larkin, Geri. *Building a Business the Buddhist Way: A Practitioner's Guidebook*. Berkeley: Celestial Arts, 1999.

————. *Tap Dancing in Zen*. Berkeley: Celestial Arts, 2000.

National Organization for Competency Assurance. "National Commission for Certifying Agencies (NCCA)." http://www.noca.org/ncca/accreditation.htm.

Pilates, Joseph, Judd Robbins, and William Miller. *Pilates' Return to Life Through Contrology*. Incline Village, NV: Presentation Dynamics, 1998.

Cornell, Camilla. "Breaking-up (with a business partner) is hard to do," *Profit Magazine*. November, 2004.

Rubin, Harriet. *Soloing: Realizing Your Life's Ambition*. New York: HarperBusiness, 1999.

Stanley, Lawrence E. "About the Name Pilates."
http://www.pilatesbodytrends.com/products/pilates/pilname.html.

United States Patent and Trademark Office. www.uspto.gov.

Wiio, Osamo A. *Wiio's Laws – and Some Others*. Espoo: Weilin + Goos, 2000.

Wood, Julia. *Relational Communication: Continuity and Change in Personal Relationships*. Belmont: Wadsworth Publishing Company, 2000.

Acknowledgment

Logokinesis Publishing was founded to create a platform for discussion among mind-body practitioners. Thank you to all the teachers who supported our projects.

Without Holly Furgason and Amy Burke, no Logokinesis project is complete. This time they not only designed (Holly) and edited (Amy) the entire book, but became co-writers as well. We love you.

In the Pilates field, I would like to express gratitude and much love to Sylvia Rohmann, Aimee McDonald, Kornelia Ritterpusch, Bridget Montague, Carolyne Anthony, Kristopher Bosch, Gerald Morigeriato, and Dane Burke—your voices are in this book. Thank you Kirsten "Schmelzi" Czastrau for being a great friend, for your patience, and for always being available to manage my teaching stints in Europe.

To the founders of Pilates corporations: Brent Anderson, thank you for your support from afar. The voices of many of your teachers that are reflected in this book embody your philosophy of love for life and the Pilates community. Colleen Craig, princess of Pilates on the Ball, thank you for your inspiration and encouragement. It means so much to me and encouraged us to go ahead with yet another book. Thank you to Lynne Johnson at Balanced Body who put *Survival Skills for Pilates Teachers* in the catalog and on the map. I am also grateful to Anoushka Boone of the PILATESfoundation® UK Ltd. for letting me teach an experimental workshop in communication for Pilates teachers.

To Nancy Hodari, Eva Powers, Lynette Rassmussen, Donna Gambino, Sophie Hunter, and all the teachers I have spoken to for peer review and feedback: Bravo!

To Dr. Doug Risner and Stephen K. Stone in the dance department at Wayne State University, thank you for supporting me.

Jim Edwards, we are grateful that you were so patient and gracious, answering a million questions about printing and publishing. I repaid you amply by arguing in

French on the Cadillac!

Finally, I was so lucky to grow up surrounded by dreamweavers. Thank you to Hans, Karin, and Bernadette Conraths, and a big smile to my late grandfather, Peter Conraths.

I will never be able to repay my husband and friend Jens Lange for all the hours that this book has caused him to spend away from his boat. On the other hand, as we were writing this book, we decided to buy land in Cuba and open a bed and breakfast with Pilates studio and sailing school as soon as Castro is open to the idea. Maybe we should send him a book?

Contact Information

Belsize Studio
Avigail Ben-Ari
5 McCrone Mews
Belsize Lane
London NW3 5BG
Phone: +44 20 7431 6223
Email: avigail@belsizestudio.com
Web: www.belsizestudio.com

Body Arts and Science International
Rael Isacowitz, MA
Founder and Director
485 E. 17th Street, Suite 650
Costa Mesa, CA 92627
USA
Phone: +1 949 574 1343
Fax: +1 949 642 8139
Email: info@basipilates.com
Web: www.basipilates.com

Body Control Pilates Group
6 Langley Street
London WC2H 9JA
United Kingdom
Phone: +44 207 379 3734
Fax: +44 207 379 7551
Web: www.bodycontrolpilates.com

The Center for Women's Fitness
Carolyne Anthony, Director
2371 Delaware Drive
Ann Arbor, MI 48103
USA
Phone: +1 734 668 4077
Web: www.thecenterforwomensfitness.com

Core Grace Pilates
Khita Whyatt
211 S. 4th Avenue, Suite 1B
Ann Arbor, MI 48104
USA
Phone: +1 734 913 9046
Web: www.coregracepilates.com

Creative Body Engineering
Philip Madrid
10109 Baldwin Ave
Albuquerque, NM 87112
USA
Phone: +1 505 332 3562

Equilibrium: Mind-Body Fitness
A STOTT PILATES™ Licensed Certification Center
Nancy Hodari, Director
Eva Powers, MA, Professor,
Wayne State University
Kim Dunleavy, MS, PT, OCS
6405 Telegraph, Building G
Bloomfield Medical Village
Bloomfield Hills, MI 48301
USA
Phone: +1 248 723 6500
Email: nancy@equilibriumstudio.com
Web: www.equilibriumstudio.com

Franklin Methode Institut
Eric Franklin, Founder
Brunnenstrasse 1
86106 Usta
Switzerland
Phone: +41 43 399 0603
Fax: +41 43 399 0604
Web: www.franklin-methode.ch

Gyrotonic Expansion System®
134 Dingmans Ct.
Dingmans Ferry, PA 18328
USA
Phone: +1 570 828 0003
Email: info@gyrotonic.com
Web: www.gyrotonic.com

Interkinetic Creative Group™
Holly Furgason
San Francisco, CA
Phone: +1 415 824 1007
Email: info@ikcgroup.com
Web: www.ikcgroup.com

McEntire Workout Method
Trent McEntire, Program Director
438 Main Street, Suite 207
Rochester, MI 48307
USA
Phone: +1 248 651 5567 or toll free +1 866 373 8600
Email: trent@mcentiremethod.com
Web: www.mcentiremethod.com

Movement Center
Aimee McDonald & Nicola Conraths-Lange
201 East Liberty Street, Suite 6
Ann Arbor, MI 48104
USA
Web: www.movement-center.com

NAMASTA—North American Studio Alliance
2313 Hastings Drive
Belmont, CA 94002
USA
Phone: +1 877 626 2782 or toll free +1 877 NAMASTA
Web: www.namasta.com

Northstar Pilates Solutions, LLC
Kristopher Bosch, Dane Burke, & Gerald Morigerato, Cofounders
3 Gates Circle
Buffalo, NY 14209
Phone: +1 716 887 5052
Web: www.northstarpilates.com

Pilates & Beyond
Elizabeth Larkam, Director
Western Athletic Clubs
One Lombard Street
San Francisco, CA 94111
USA
Phone: +1 415 901 9310
Email: elarkam@wac-clubs.com

Pilates Forms
Sylvia Rohmann
Brahmsallee 16
20144 Hamburg
Germany
Email: sylvia.rohmann@freenet.de

PILATESfoundation® UK Limited
Anoushka Boone
P.O. Box 36052
London SW16 1XQ
 Phone: +44 7071 781 859
Fax: +44 20 8696 0088
 Web: www.pilatesfoundation.com

Pilates Method Alliance
P.O.Box 370906
Miami, FL 33137
USA
Phone: +1 866 573 4945
Fax: +1 305 573 4461
Email: info@pilatesmethodalliance.org
Web: www.pilatesmethodalliance.org

Polestar Pilates Education, LLC
International Headquarters
12380 SW 82 Avenue
Miami, FL 33156
USA
Phone: +1 305 666 0037 or toll free +1 800 387 3651
Web: www.polestarpilates.com

Lynnette Rasmussen, OTR
Case Manager/Pilates Instructor
University of Michigan Spine Program
325 E. Eisenhower Parkway
Suite 100
Ann Arbor, MI 48108
Phone: +1 734 615 1744

Owen Seitel
Idell Berman Seitel & Rutchik, LLP
465 California Street, Suite 300
San Francisco, CA 94104
USA
Phone:+1 415 986 2400
Email: owen.seitel@ibslaw.com
Web: www.ibsrlaw.com

STOTT PILATES™* Merrithew Corporation
Lindsay G. Merrithew & Moira Merrithew, Cofounders
2200 Yonge Street, Suite 500
Toronto, ON M4S 2C6
Canada
Phone: +1 416 482 4050 or toll free +1 800 910 0001
Fax: +1 416 482 2742
Email: info@stottpilates.com
Web: www.stottpilates.com

Studio für Körperbewusstsein
Kornelia Ritterpusch
Grindelhof 89, Hs.9, Garten
20146 Hamburg
Germany
Phone: +49 40 410 7273
Fax: +49 404 136 3417
Email: kornelia@studiofurkorperbewusstsein.de

Logokinesis™ offers more than just books. Nicola Conraths-Lange and Jens Lange teach and offer consultation to Pilates teachers and studio owners around the world. Contact us directly to set up an appointment or to schedule a speaking or teaching engagement at your event.

Logokinesis Publishing

If there is a book in you, we would like to hear about it! We often collaborate with practitioners, movement teachers, and musicians.
Please direct inquiries to info@logokinesis.com.

Logokinesis Education Workshops

Information on workshops for Pilates and dance can be found at www.logokinesis. com. You can also contact Nicola directly at nicola@logokinesis.com.

Logokinesis Consulting

Jens Lange offers consulting for aspiring and established studio owners. Phone consultations are by appointment and typically last 1 hour.
You can contact Jens directly at jens@logokinesis.com.

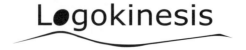

Order Form

Logokinesis Publishing
805 Third Street
Ann Arbor, MI 48103
USA

Please ship order to:

Name

Address

City, State, Zip

Country

I would like to order the following titles:

........Copies: *Survival Skills for Pilates Teachers*   @ $24.95 = ...

........Copies: *Pilates Space*   @ $39.95 = ...

+ Shipping & Handling @ $7.00

Total: ....

Please enclose a check or money order made out to "Logokinesis" in US$.